ETHICS FROM THE GROUND UP

ETHICS FROM THE GROUND UP

EMERGING DEBATES, CHANGING PRACTICES AND NEW VOICES IN HEALTHCARE

EDITORS: J. WINTRUP, H. BIGGS,
T. BRANNELLY, A. FENWICK, R. INGHAM
AND D. WOODS

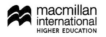 macmillan
international
HIGHER EDUCATION

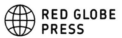 RED GLOBE
PRESS

First published 2019 by
RED GLOBE PRESS

Red Globe Press in the UK is an imprint of Springer Nature Limited, registered
in England, company number 785998, of 4 Crinan Street,
London, N1 9XW.

Red Globe Press® is a registered trademark in the United States,
the United Kingdom, Europe and other countries.

ISBN 978–1–352–00275–1

This book is printed on paper suitable for recycling and made from fully
managed and sustained forest sources. Logging, pulping and manufacturing
processes are expected to conform to the environmental regulations of the
country of origin.

A catalogue record for this book is available from the British Library.

A catalog record for this book is available from the Library of Congress.

For Eloise Megan Land

Every day her generous, courageous, loyal and beautiful self

CONTENTS

FOREWORD

Suzanne Shale

What does doing 'everyday ethics' mean for healthcare practitioners?

This is an example of a day-to-day dilemma that will be familiar to many.[1]

> Eric is a 72-year-old man who was diagnosed with colorectal cancer at the age of 70. He has been treated by radiotherapy, surgery and a temporary ileostomy. He has just had the ileostomy reversed and was expecting a hospital stay of two or three days. Unfortunately, it took some time for his bowel to start functioning again, and since it did he has been experiencing distressing, frequent and violent attacks of diarrhoea. He has now been in hospital for eight days.
>
> Eric is the type of patient who tries to put a brave face on things, and tends to joke around with his consultant, the foundation doctors and nursing staff. But you got to know Eric well when he first had a stoma, and he is a bit more honest with you when you stop by to see him. 'My tail end is so sore' he tells you. 'I can't sit; I can't lie on my back – it is really painful. I seem to have no control over my bowel now. It's just awful. But I'm desperate to go home; my friends can't feed the cats forever. I said that to the doctors. The hospital is so busy, I don't think I ought to stay here if I can be at home.'
>
> The youngest survivor of several siblings, Eric doesn't have any close family. He lives alone in a rather out-of-the-way cottage he bought with his partner, Frank, who died two years ago. They were intending to do it up but ran out of money. You know it has no central heating and that the tiny bathroom has six steps leading up to it. All winter the hospital has been running at close to 100 per cent bed occupancy.

---

[1] It was first developed to stimulate discussion among practitioners working with Macmillan Cancer Support, who recognise it as immediately relevant to their concerns.

Having heard from the doctors treating him, the bed manager is of a view that, despite the continuing diarrhoea and his general frailty, Eric is medically fit for discharge. You cannot imagine how Eric will cope with the minimal support that can be offered by community-based services. What ethical issues does this raise for you?

One of my favourite ways of starting a study day or conference or meeting with care professionals is to ask them to talk about what gave them the greatest satisfaction in their last week at work. After a common initial reaction – that the entire week has been an unmitigated disaster and they can't think of anything about it that was remotely good – and given permission to reflect on the whole past month if necessary, a moving conversation ensues. Three themes frequently emerge: (i) the delight in seeing a patient, or someone important to the patient, getting a benefit from something you have done for them; (ii) the pleasure in drawing on your expertise, and using it to good effect; and (iii) the gratification to be found in relationships with colleagues, perhaps those whom you have helped, or who assisted you, or a colleague with whom you have had a better than expected interaction. When we then move on to discussing the ethical challenges that paid caregivers encounter in their work, we discover that they often threaten to disrupt these important sources of fulfilment.

Eric's unenviable situation doesn't present professionals with an ethical dilemma because it is new, unusual, or requires special ethical expertise. Quite the opposite. It happens frequently in a care system running at full capacity, is immediately recognisable, and contributes to the day-to-day moral distress that can accompany care work. (Pauly and colleagues have examined the various meanings attributed to the term *moral distress*: centrally, it refers to the feelings that arise from 'difficulties navigating practice while upholding professional values, responsibilities and duties' (Pauly et al., 2012). For me, this scenario is an 'ethical' one because it goes directly to Bernard Williams' question, 'how should one live?'(Williams, 1985). And it presents a 'dilemma' because bringing it to a satisfactory conclusion will require both careful scrutiny of different parties' interests, and also the exercise of great skill in negotiating the outcome.

Moreover, Eric's situation severely tests all three of the cherished motivations: doing good, being an expert and getting on with colleagues. The resources to do good appear to be unavailable (and frustratingly, if Eric is sent home and suffers harm, it will undo much of the good that has already been done). Being an expert hasn't necessarily helped. This practitioner's expert assessment differs from that of her colleagues (whether this puts her in an awkward situation depends on whether the team she works with values hearing different views). But unless she can do something about Eric's situation, the expert listening that elicited his doubts and anxieties merely serves to accentuate her difficulties. And finally, there is her interaction with the bed manager to worry about. Each of them has a different focus, the practitioner mindful of Eric's well-being and the bed manager mindful of the population of patients waiting for a bed. Whether this different focus turns into a conflict depends on how well they manage their interaction.

What is the everyday ethical expertise that the practitioner will need to call upon here? It is both epistemic and performative (Weinstein, 1993, 1994). First, there is the epistemic expertise: she must draw on her ability to make a clinical assessment (including Eric's psychosocial needs and the risk of harm to him) and appreciate the implications; but she must also be able to explain and justify her assessment to her colleagues. Next is the performative expertise: she will need the know-how and skill to navigate the system, to have a constructive negotiation with colleagues, to change the bed manager's mind to prioritise Eric or change her own mind to prioritise other patients' claims, and to do all of this in a timely fashion. Further elements will be necessary to sustain her. She will need the emotional expertise to manage her own response to the situation and to deal with the residue of distress she may feel if things don't go Eric's way. Perhaps she will seek guidance, wondering what a real expert would do in these circumstances. (But who is she to ask?[2])

This collection is concerned with 'surfacing the ethical issues implicit in everyday health and care, and in exploring the questions and concerns that emerge' (page xii). The opportunity to do so is vital. Only through attending to the reality of everyday ethics in care work will we come to understand its challenges; comprehend the nature of the expertise that enables such challenges to be overcome by professionals seeking to realise citizens' interests; and begin to appreciate what we need to do to sustain care professionals in ethically demanding roles. And it is by attending to the voices of those less heard in ethical texts – as we have the opportunity to do in the third part of this collection – that we come to realise the intimate connections that exist between professionals, learners and citizens in the care enterprise. The diversity of issues and of voices captured in this collection enriches our approach to the question of how we should live, not just as professionals but as fellow human beings.

---

2 See also L.M. Rasmussen (ed.). (2005) *Ethics Expertise: History, Contemporary Perspectives, and Applications*, Dordrecht: Springer; M. Cholbi (2007) Moral expertise and the credentials problem, *Ethical Theory & Moral Practice*, 10, 323–34.

Bibliography

Cholbi, M. (2007) Moral expertise and the credentials problem. *Ethical Theory & Moral Practice*, 10, pp. 323–34.

Pauly, B.M., Varcoe, C. and Storch, J. (2012) Framing the issues: moral distress in healthcare. *Hec Forum*, 24, 1–11.

Rasmussen, L.M. (ed.). (2005) *Ethics Expertise: History, Contemporary Perspectives, and Applications*. Dordrecht: Springer.

Weinstein, B.D. (1993) What is an expert? *Theoretical Medicine*, 14, pp. 57–73.

Weinstein, B.D. (1994) The possibility of ethical expertise. *Theoretical Medicine*, 15, pp. 61–75.

Williams, B. (1985) *Ethics and the Limits of Philosophy*. London: Fontana Paperbacks and William Collins.

INTRODUCTION

Julie Wintrup

Exploring ethics from the ground up

The purpose of this collection is to introduce new ways of thinking about healthcare work as a moral and collective endeavour. It is part of a wider initiative to explore the ethics of everyday health and care that includes dedicated conferences (e.g. On Everyday Ethics, 2016[3]) and draws on the work of practitioners who write and blog (see, e.g., Tomlinson, 2018[4]). A group of contributors go on to explore more explicitly theoretical perspectives in the chapters that follow, each sparked by experiences, conversations, analysis and research. The collection examines ethical work, both practice and policy, that is often tacit in nature, what Lambek (2010, p. 2) describes as 'grounded in agreement rather than rule, in practice rather than knowledge or belief, and happening without calling undue attention to itself'. Although chapters differ in style and focus, they share the educational goal of surfacing the ethical issues implicit in everyday health and care, and in exploring the questions and concerns that emerge. Such close analysis tends to raise new and even more difficult issues, which seems at odds with the urge to find answers and resolutions and can be experienced – in particular by those who feel unfamiliar with ethical concepts or outside decision-making arenas – as frustrating and even deskilling. However, we propose that realising complexity *and* seeking answers are the central elements of ethical reasoning. Dewey (1910, p. 12) described the 'demand for the solution of a perplexity' as the 'steadying' factor that provokes learning. In other words, and to summarise our educational stance: *not* knowing, being open to new information, indeed being prepared to be more perplexed, while remaining committed to seeking solutions, however imperfect, is the basis of learning healthcare ethics. Such learning occurs when working with and learning from other

---

[3] Everyday ethical dilemmas in healthcare: power, politics and practices, http://2016.oneverydayethics.co.uk/.

[4] Jonathon Tomlinson, A better NHS: exploring the relationships between doctors and patients and health policy, https://abetternhs.net/about/.

people, in unique situations and during testing times, and with the people and in the places they live and manage health conditions. Chapter authors, in very different ways, offer their own experiences of not knowing, questioning, and using ethical concepts to generate and appraise ways forward.

Although this is not a book that *begins* with moral philosophy, thinking philosophically is encouraged throughout and is necessary to get the most from several chapters. It purposely offers alternative routes into foundational ethical theories, offering the interested beginner and those more familiar with the subject opportunities to examine and critique some taken-for-granted health and education practices. It does not compartmentalise 'types' of ethics or promote specific concepts such as biomedical, legal or research ethics, and it does not foreground policy, procedures, rules or professional codes – although those are variously discussed in contextual terms. Neither is it following in the tradition of disciplinary-based 'ethics for *x*', *x* denoting whichever professional group is the intended audience. This is because many texts already cover those narrower interests more than adequately, and though the collection reflects authors' specialist interests, our purpose in writing this book is different. It is designed to be of broad interest and accessible to the non-specialist, including students, practitioners, people using services, health educators, managers and interested others. Chapter topics are diverse, our hope being that interests are piqued in new readers who associate health-care ethics only with more traditional medical decision-making.

Our intention is first and foremost to shine a light on the tricky, sometimes ambiguous, almost always contingent circumstances that healthcare work requires of us every day: if this, then maybe that, but possibly the other – or neither. Problems that do not have easy solutions prompt deeper reflection and discussion, often (but possibly, not often enough) in the midst of action. They require flexibility and cooperation among and beyond professional clinical and care teams. Such rich, organic learning is by its nature contextual and dynamic, because 'what it does is continually alter the context in which it occurs' rather than simply alter the properties of the learner, as Beckett and Hager (2002, p. 146) describe. Yet broadening the scope of ethical work, from a care or treatment decision to managerial or political decisions, a lifestyle choice or sharing of risk, raises new ethical issues. For example, when alliances break down – between patient and health professionals, or among different disciplines within a team – divisions can develop and over time become entrenched. Distrust and feelings of betrayal may have damaging effects far beyond the immediate circle of people involved. In public discourse, we hear relatively little about successful day-to-day healthcare work with its negotiated solutions and compromises, because in general this remains private and between individuals, and in most countries is protected by law. So our impression of ethical dilemmas is often shaped by the out-of-the-ordinary situations that also become known about and debated in the media, meaning newspaper editors or those with the greatest social media reach determine their framing. Many voices are drowned out in such arenas. Others cannot or choose not to speak, leaving us to speculate on how situations may have arisen or why judgements were made. In bringing this collection together, we seek to learn more about the many kinds of ethical work from voices rarely heard and alternative vantage points. Schön (1987, p. 3) memorably described 'the swampy lowlands, where situations are confusing messes incapable of technical solution and usually involve problems of greatest human concern', reflecting the messy, intimate, routine nature of health practice, where learning and change may be uncomfortable, traumatic even, and may leave emotional scars. So a central message of the book is that we need to work together to better understand the range of factors that enable ethical reasoning and evaluation to take place in imperfect realities, and we begin by examining experience. Such an examination crosses the practice and classroom divide. It acknowledges the problems with terminology and requires inclusive language, detailed description and perspective taking. It obliges us to rehearse and articulate new and often complicated ideas, and to struggle with conflicting goals. Bringing together a collection that describes many kinds of experiences is a step towards redrawing the boundaries of healthcare ethics and extending its scope of interest.

How might such diverse perspectives contribute to health education and practice?

It is our contention that people involved in the work of healthcare – by which we mean not only the workforce but also unpaid and precariously employed carers, and those who work every day managing long-term conditions, disabilities or illness – are part of realising and relating 'the ethical', in their relationships, actions and stories. Sometimes this will be cultivated in teams or families, or through training, or in the intimate and intersubjective spaces between carer and cared-for. Although it is unlikely to be articulated in philosophical terms or even thought through in more abstract, intellectual ways, concerns may centre on such things as fairness, kindness or, more recently, the ubiquitous notion of 'compassion'. Bringing together a range of perspectives, although a small step in a continuous project, is part of beginning to broaden what we think of as ethical care. Yet more perspectives are sorely needed; Ion et al. (2018, p. 99) assert 'the ability to work with complexity, ambiguity and uncertainty in a culturally safe way may require considering ethical frameworks from other locations if we are to avoid the pitfall of assuming that the common ethical frameworks of Western Europe and North America make sense to populations whose belief systems were forged elsewhere'. Without expanding the scope of health and care ethics, we risk debating moral issues only in the midst, and heat, of crisis, from the more established points of view, and then in terms decided by those who may have a specific agenda. In the same spirit, we advocate moving on from understanding ethics as a top-down application of principles, or as a system of calculating uncertain future risks and benefits, often known as applied ethics. Such approaches, Lawlor (2007) asserts, do not serve those in health education programmes well, much less offer scope for a more inclusive approach. He suggests such abstractions may unwittingly alienate students who may otherwise have a lively interest in more philosophically oriented topics.

The project we are calling 'ethics from the ground up' is intended to engage, to spark an interest in the areas of health practice that are often out of sight or just seem too difficult, and to introduce the new kinds of questions posed by the ways we live our lives, in often imperfect circumstances and contradictory ways. The main interest throughout is in the ethical as encountered and described by people whose lives, work, families and interests are intertwined with healthcare in different ways. This is important for Tronto (1993, p. 178) because for her, the *doing* of ethical work is where ideas and dispositions become part of moral conduct, because 'people must engage in both private and public practices that teach them, and reinforce their senses of, these moral concerns'. In a similar vein, Zacka (2017, p. 35) explores the importance of discretion in transforming policy intentions, by those working directly with people in receipt of public services, asking 'how street-level bureaucrats inhabit these spaces of discretion, how they negotiate compromises among the plurality of goals and values they must remain sensitive to, and how they find the resources to do so in an environment that often makes good moral judgement remarkably difficult'. Our starting point, then, is not how to reach a decision in a given situation through mental reasoning processes, or by examining in detached and dispassionate ways the 'hard cases'. We begin with the goals of seeking to recognise and become attuned to the moral aspects of everyday care while in the moment; of questioning and investigating the environmental influences that inform our actions and decisions in and beyond the personal encounter; and of realising the part played by the exercising of discretion and moral agency. By framing our goals in such a way, not only does the familiar become more interesting – and in a fruitful way, more perplexing – but develops ways of thinking in preparation for more testing situations ahead.

Such a questioning, receptive disposition is only the beginning, however, of a necessary but far from sufficient attribute to cultivate. For Rest (in Bebeau, 2010) four developmental steps are involved: sensitivity, judgement, motivation and commitment to action, each of which develops over time and through practice. But progress may not be smooth or unidirectional – as the authors show in the chapters that follow, emotions provoked by unsettling events are sometimes repressed, justified or trivialised in some way, or we may seem to take a step backwards following a difficult experience. Developing judgement when alternatives are uncertain, and remaining motivated and committed in the face of opposition or a lack of resources, cannot be taken for granted simply as a feature of qualifications or experience. So the notion of ethics from the ground up has meaning in terms of beginning with what is in front of us: the people and places we know, the things that happen around us in familiar procedures and taken for granted routines, and with the unspoken and under-explored aspects of those common experiences. The book invites us to shine a light on less well-examined practices, debates and voices to learn more about their ethical aspects and implications for care.

But the notion of ethics being 'ground up' is not simply about 'understanding the ethical issues occurring at ground level' – it is a much bigger project. The expression was first used by Richard Ashcroft, at a conference dedicated to the ethics of the everyday, to describe an empirical approach to researching healthcare as a practice that aims to be, and is required to be, consistent with certain values and commitments. For Dewey (1910), such empiricism was central to experiential and experimental learning. In the UK, at its inception in 1948, the National Health Service (NHS) was founded on three core principles: that healthcare meets the needs of everyone, is free at the point of delivery and is based on clinical need, not the ability to pay (Delamothe, 2008). These were expanded recently to include, among other things, placing 'the patient at the heart of everything', best value and accountability to communities and patients (The Department of Health, 2015). Meanwhile, inquiries into failures or poor standards in healthcare reiterate the importance of a healthcare system founded on fairness, openness and equal treatment. Francis (2013) went further, asserting throughout his inquiry report into Mid Staffordshire Hospital that staff should put patients' interests *before their own*. Indeed the government accepted this recommendation, stating that the expectation 'staff put patients before themselves' (Department of Health, 2015) ought to be enshrined in the NHS Constitution. Research into 'resilience' does not find such self-sacrifice to be necessary or advisable, however, and care for self is seen as central to responsible, sustainable practice: 'Doctors need to be able to care for themselves in order to offer the best care to their patients' (Howe et al., 2012, p. 350). Similarly ideological stances are reflected in codes of professional conduct, which describe the ideal of the good professional. So given the plethora of explicit and detailed ethical principles embedded in policy, law and subsequently in commissioning guidance, an empirical approach to an ethics from the ground up might set itself the goal of discovering how such high standards, robust principles and commitments to action are manifested not only in professional behaviours but in every aspect of care and treatment. Whether at the bedside or homeless people's shelter, in the boardroom or purchasing department, or in local and national political arenas, actions and decisions have moral antecedents and implications. An empirical approach invites us to begin to formulate research questions and consider methodological approaches, to consider what would constitute data and to seek a wide and diverse audience for findings. It would necessitate confronting the less visible effects of social behaviours and power imbalances; not only those we associate with traditional hierarchies or doctor–patient divides, but those exercised between and within workforce groups, or constituted through access to forms of knowledge or representation, or generated by informal networks and interest groups.

Where does ethics from the ground up take us?

In this book, we encourage healthcare education to embrace an interdisciplinary, patient and service user-led approach to constructing ethics as a shared set of interests, in which tacit knowledge and the expertise of lived experience sits alongside disciplinary and technical forms of expertise. In such a construction of the ethical, 'roles' are less important than contribution. Individuals bring multiple perspectives and different insights to ethical dilemmas or problems and are encouraged to discover and explore others' views and priorities. Emotion, often seen as anathema to cool reasoning, is viewed as intrinsic to the human conditions that prompt ethical debate: injustices, vulnerability and life-and-death decisions. Concepts such as compassion and resilience are understood to be contingent, situated and emotional in quality.

   Healthcare ethics, once firmly within the ivory tower of medical academia, is gradually being democratised. People take an interest in individual dilemmas shared publicly or in blogs, engaging radio programmes, documentaries and dramas look in detail at individual stories, and networks and communities use social media to open up debate. At the same time, new risks to privacy and confidentiality are posed by new ways of communicating. As things change and evolve, what is or is not ethical is far from settled. Doctors using social messaging services to communicate patient information are breaking privacy laws, yet when understood as part of a life-saving intervention to perform surgery or in the context of the total shutdown of a network, such a response seems a rational, creative and even praiseworthy solution to a crisis. Beginning to think about *who decides* what constitutes the ethical is an exercise that invites us to think philosophically and so is a fitting place to begin a book that starts with the everyday work of healthcare. Such work requires that we think not only about the way we make decisions, or resource, organise and regulate health services, but also about ways to live our lives, and to respond to one another's needs.

It seems then that the concept of healthcare ethics as a somewhat dry and abstract topic is out of step with society. When courts of law are asked to decide between medical recommendations and a request to be assisted to die, or to access an experimental therapy, people across all sectors of society get involved; they discuss life-and-death issues in the workplace and on Facebook, and form opinions. Treatment and technological advancements mean new kinds of decisions have to be made by people using health services, often in cooperation with professionals, with those responsible for purchasing and commissioning services, and sometimes with numerous others. Often such decisions threaten a person's privacy or necessitate the sharing of familial knowledge, or need to be revisited throughout the course of a lifelong disorder or disability. Choices may involve imperfect predictions, incomplete information and complicated data, and answers may well be temporary or provisional. Ethics is no longer, if it ever was, the preserve of health professionals.

Why is the notion of ground-up ethics a stimulus for learning?

If the traditional idea of healthcare ethics is shaped by situations that arise in the public domain, the kinds of questions that arise in more private domains remain under-explored. Their importance is overlooked until, as happens for some, the issues become public, or those involved come to view them as morally problematic or important to share with others. As a result, we tend to learn about and from healthcare problems that become public. These tend to be rare and unusual – such as the separation of conjoined twins when one is bound to die from the operation, or a dispute between patient and doctor that has reached the law courts. This public–private dimension is not binary, but a continuum, and to a degree subjective. So this is by no means suggested as a fixed category, but rather a loose and functional distinction. Those in the public arena, as in the examples above, tend to be high stakes, life-or-death decisions, reported in real time and generating boundless levels of interest and emotion. When what is at stake is how well someone is able to access (say) a form of therapy that will improve their quality of life but is not essential to live, the issue might seem to be on a different continuum; with life-or-death outcomes at one end, and routine, everyday health (and social) care needs at the other. Like the public–private continuum, situations may change and move between higher or lower stakes. Finding a new heart for a gravely ill 20-year-old may move from high life-or-death stakes after a successful transplant, to low stakes, everyday care when the cost of transport to a specialist unit 60 miles away has to be compared with paying for essential prescriptions, meaning one or the other may have to be forfeited.

Viewed in this way, it is possible to see a relationship between the way ethical or moral questions in healthcare and in social care simultaneously shape and are shaped by the 'high stakes or public' quadrant of these two spectrums. Private encounters are, necessarily, between individuals entitled to and obliged to respect privacy. Low stakes issues attract little attention, until or unless they become high stakes. The extraordinary, or the highly emotive, seems to elicit empathy, and so we risk overlooking the moral problems inherent in the private or routine aspects of healthcare. Yet because this is where we tend to work together, cooperatively most of the time, the ordinary has untapped potential for learning, as we appreciate one another's priorities and sensitivities. Relationships, particularly those that are outside of the normal run of things, and the daily routines and sustaining features of lives, offer rich learning that might better prepare us as ethical social beings, for the high stakes or public encounters when they come along.

This book is interested in the variety of experiences that we can understand to have ethical dimensions. It offers insights into how awareness of ethical concerns is heightened and into the process of becoming familiar with the moral components of situations, rather than seeing problems as puzzles to be solved or arguments to be won. Most importantly, it directs our gaze to aspects of healthcare that have been neglected in more traditional biomedico-legal constructions of the ethical.

The structure of the book

It is helpful to consider how this text might be used, whether in formal ethics education by students and by educators, or to deepen and broaden a more general interest in healthcare ethics. The three parts may be approached sequentially, offering a breadth of perspective and a diversity of theoretical frameworks, and requiring different kinds of intellectual work. We would like to think too that chapters might be selected individually and read as essays on a particular theme, standing alone as a meaningful contribution to ethical debate. The three commentaries at the end of Parts 1, 2 and 3 are deliberately unstructured and reflective, drawing out some connecting themes and posing further questions for exploration. We trust there will be many more connections to be made, and very different questions, reflections and ideas ignited, in the minds of individual readers and (ideally) in practice and classroom-based discussion groups. Although there is no expectation of prior formal philosophical training, particular chapters lend themselves to further interpretation of the language of ethics and a broader understanding of key theories. However, some experience of, and a deep interest in, care and treatment provision is an important prerequisite. We resisted the temptation to summarise chapters in overly directive or reductive ways, in keeping with our central message that each of us will bring unanticipated, unique insights to chapters, all of equal value. Indeed, a well-facilitated, free-ranging, student-led discussion – or as Pardales and Girod (2006, p. 304) describe, 'following the inquiry where it leads' – is recommended.

Although the contributions differ from one another in style, approach and intention, each offers a novel perspective inviting ways to glimpse ethical underpinnings in what might otherwise be viewed as somewhat dry organisational, clinical or political concerns. Authors include a poet, health researchers, experts by experience, students, health bloggers, health professionals and academics in law, philosophy, sociology, primary care, psychology and health sciences, all interested in expanding ways to define and scrutinise the moral aspects of healthcare. Some authors begin with the personal and the specific, going on to illuminate more general ethical considerations, whereas others begin by raising compelling questions for both new and familiar practices.

Interspersed between sections, poetry by nurse and spoken word poet Molly Case offers an evocative, analytical critique of the everyday work of nursing care, often taking place in less than ideal conditions. Molly's caring goes beyond caregiving; it sees much and is observant, often revealing uncomfortable and troubling insights. The ethical work of nursing is firmly behind the curtain, yet ever present. 'The Last 1000 Days' – following in a tradition of poems written to nurses – dares us to value the last days of a life one iota less than any other days in any other lives. In 'Better Than This', raw anger is jarring; the line 'fake feelings to disguise underhand dealings' has meaning well beyond health services. In the final two poems, Molly is still the student nurse. Her famous 'Nursing the Nation' shares the minutiae of nursing care while 'roaring' against the castigations of those who know nothing of it. We end with 'Welcome to Paradise', non-traditional in structure and compelling in its immediacy. The first day of placement – so familiar to many of us that the nervousness is infectious – and it is the trivia of the everyday that stays long after reading; mashing potato into soup, snatches of conversation, endless daytime television, questions left unasked. It is not by accident that we close the book with a welcome, imperfect as this paradise might be.

Part 1 introduces what we are calling emerging debates in healthcare ethics. In the first chapter, Engward and Papanikitas offer the 'invisible' ethics of inter disciplinarity as an under-explored concept, highlighting the unique ethical challenges faced by the wider healthcare team. They question the utility of traditional inter disciplinary education with its tendency to make assumptions about shared values, while underplaying the very real tensions that exist between professions and specialisms, with their different traditions, responsibilities and purposes. Raising questions ultimately about patient safety and healthcare quality, they make a compelling case for a better, more empirically based investigation into the ethics of inter disciplinary working. Brannelly continues this theme, presenting empirical research that surfaces hidden practices in an area of health provision she describes as private, not visible or known to those outside it. Her analysis of mental health provision that includes 'protection' – a term she problematises – invites a radical rethink of how services might more effectively promote equality for groups already marginalised. Brannelly offers the framework of the ethics of care, with its focus on moral action and its commitment to justice and politics, as a source of enlightenment and renewal. The final chapter in Part 1 resonates with the idea of ethics as hidden. Brown examines the ways we seek to hide our inner psychic distress as healthcare students and academics, in order to maintain a pretence that we do not have mental health difficulties, instead asking people who use mental health services to expose themselves on our behalf. In a subtle and nuanced discussion, Brown navigates the liminal as she questions how we might resist, at one extreme, the polarising 'us and them' discourse that silence risks, and at the other, what she calls a 'large-scale confessional'. Raising ethical and pedagogic issues, Brown notes that we ask students simultaneously to use the self therapeutically in their practice while denying aspects of the self in keeping with notions of professional boundaries. Woods and Ingham close Part 1, drawing out themes from chapters that highlight the threat to ethical and high-quality care posed by a focus on such things as efficiency, measurement and output, at the cost of reflection on its real purpose and the part played by human relationships.

Part 2 challenges the kinds of practices and philosophies typically explored in healthcare ethics, beginning with Dowling's fascinating exploration of the ethical issues raised by breastmilk sharing and donation. In a historically and culturally informed discussion, she asks such questions as these: is giving milk different to giving blood? And if the means are there to share, why would society seek to regulate women's gift of milk to other women? In another provoking piece, Engward gives an overview of the ethical implications of the military covenant that differentiates between *soldiers* – those able to be deployed – and *patients*, ex-military personnel in need of treatment, who for health reasons are no longer able to be deployed. She unpacks the historical and instrumental reasoning behind methods of categorising and prioritising need, exposing many contradictory and often unfathomable practices, going on to clarify what might be a more sustainable and ethically defensible stance by the state. The third chapter of Part 2 presents empirical research into the reasoning and decision-making of paediatricians when end-of-life best interests decisions are made for children with severe disabilities. Picton-Howell also draws on research into parents' experiences of such decisions and explores the kinds of disagreements that take place. She goes on to appraise the place ethical guidance provided to paediatricians plays in resolving such disagreement when the interests of children, parents and doctors are considered. Biggs and Fenwick conclude Part 2 by extending the ideas introduced by the chapter authors, questioning the distinction between private and public arenas and reminding us of the state's responsibilities towards society as well as designated groups. They introduce cross-cutting ethical concepts that offer ways to better understand how these kinds of concerns are pertinent to healthcare provision more broadly.

Part 3 gives voice to those least heard in ethics texts, with honest and painful accounts of the struggle to remain sensitive to distress and yet buoyant enough to survive. In the first chapter of Part 3, Hogue and Ennis-O'Connor call for a rethink of research ethics processes that have failed to keep up with social and technological change. As health bloggers and leaders in international social networking, they offer a unique critique of the casual use of blogs and other forms of social media by the health research community. They offer questions to prompt a more thoughtful approach to, among other things, the meaning of informed consent and the importance of context. Stenning, in conversation with Wintrup, develops the themes of identity, equality and power, as a co-producer of healthcare working from the perspective of experience. His call for fair reward for equal work is contextualised in the complicated and, for many, deeply anxiety-provoking benefits assessment system that all too often prevents a re-entry into paid work. Stenning has recommendations for employers who want to work fairly and creatively with people using services, while reminding us of the many obstacles. Finally, Dunne offers another personal and at times painful account, this time from the experience of being a medical student. Redolent of many points made in the poems of Case, by Stenning, and in Part 2 by Brown, Dunne describes being a novice and, because of that, in many ways an outsider. She reminds us just how much is taken for granted and is at risk when we fail to recognise the everyday ethical problems that infuse healthcare, or seem to separate those problems from more abstract philosophical classroom discussions. Her embodied account is at times hard to read, yet offers a timely reminder that even the most routine healthcare work – taking blood, learning up-to-date techniques – is an intrinsically moral pursuit that places demands upon us.

Brannelly's summation of these chapters, and closing reflection, focuses on a central thread of 'the real' as it is experienced and as it connects to philosophical deliberation. Among other insights, she contrasts the compelling words of authors in Part 3 with those of more legalistic, detached ethical proclamations such as professional codes. Urging everyday language if we are to work together more fruitfully, Brannelly brings us to the central questions of how to share power without avoiding responsibility, and how to remain both resilient and vulnerable as we move between uncertainty and action. Offering insights from care ethics, she concludes that understanding the ethics of the everyday humanises healthcare, connecting the personal with the political in direct and meaningful ways.

References

Ballatt, J. and Campling, P. (2011) *Intelligent Kindness: Reforming the Culture of Healthcare*. London: Royal College of Psychiatrists.

Carel, H. (2008) *Illness: The Art of Living*. Durham: Acumen.

Bebeau, M. (2010) The defining issues test and the four component model: Contributions to professional education. *Journal of Moral Education*, 31(3), pp. 271–95.

Beckett, D. and Hager, P. (2002) *Life, Work and Learning: Practice in Postmodernity*. London: Routledge.

Delamothe, T. (2008) Founding principles. *British Medical Journal*, 336, p. 1216.

Department of Health (2015) The NHS constitution for England. https://www.gov.uk/government/publications/the-nhs-constitution-for-england/the-nhs-constitution-for-england (accessed 16 September 2017).

Dewey, J. (1910) *How We Think*. Boston, MA: D.C. Heath and Co.

Francis, R. (2013) *Report of the Mid Staffordshire NHS Foundation Trust Public Inquiry*. London: The Stationery Office.

Howe, A., Smajdor, A. and Stockl, A. (2012) Towards an understanding of resilience and its relevance to medical training. *Medical Education*, 46(4), pp. 349–56.

Ion, R., DeSouza, R. and Kerin, T. (2018) Teaching ethics: intersectionality, care failure and moral courage. *Nurse Education Today*, 61, pp. 98–100.

Lambek, M. (2010) *Ordinary Ethics: Anthropology, Language, and Action*. New York: Fordham University Press.

Lawlor, R. (2007) Moral theories in teaching applied ethics. *Journal of Medical Ethics*, 33(6), pp. 370–72.

Pardales, M. and Girod, M. (2006) Community of inquiry: its past and present future. *Educational Philosophy and Theory*, 38(3), pp. 299–309.

Schön, D. (1987) *Educating the Reflective Practitioner*. New York: Basic Book.

Zacka, B. (2017) *When the State Meets the Street*. London: Harvard University Press.

PART 1

Emerging Debates

The Last 1000 Days[1,2]

Molly Case

These days slip away like coins into a slot.
I sit here; the person, the life,
the woman that time forgot.
Caught between hospital bays
and grey rooms that speak
nothing of the life I've had.

These days, these days,
always in my memory;
Post Office and tea dance reverie.
But recently, hazy
as hospital wards become mazes,
and I am amazed
at all the ways I am lost
when once I was so found.

When we kissed so hard
we felt the ground move,
these days,
spent on the windswept,
salt-slapped dunes by the bay.

---

[1] This poem was inspired by Professor Brian Dolan's research into perceiving time as the most important currency in healthcare. As healthcare workers, how can we ensure that time isn't wasted when people come into hospital? How can we speed things up? How can we make sure that we truly understand that the time people have in their last days is just as precious as all the days that have come before? MC

These days that seemed to go on
until the horizon line,
where the sea, the sun
and the moon aligned
and we were just part of it
and we danced in the shallows
that had never felt so cold.
Until now, because these blankets are thin
and my skin has not felt your warm palms
in years.

In here kind faces come and go
but the wait spreads out,
slow and unknowable ahead
these days are spent staring at walls
and lying in bed.

Today they say an investigation is needed:
why your heart is filling with water.
A wheelchair comes, another hospital porter
who whistles old Nat King Cole songs
and I sing along,
all of the words that once made me strong.
These days, these days
that now all blur into one.

But then a nurse comes in and says:
Hello, my name is Kate
and together we're going to get you home soon.
I think of the dunes, the moon, and you
forever framed photographs in my front room,
soon to be back again,
as Kate goes on to explain:

We'll get this referral sped up
the results of the scan on the way
so that you don't have to waste
any more time sitting here today
these days are yours
that we must help look after
let's see if we can get your medication
ordered just a little bit faster.

The staff are remarkable,
always here with me
yet all so busy
I wonder if they forget
I don't have all the time in the world –
though I'm not leaving yet!
But today something has shifted,
no longer the woman
that spends time in bed:
my life is a horizon line
still unfurling out ahead.

And it leads me
home to my garden,
'When I Fall in Love' drifts
down the path
a single sparrow flies past
sits on the ledge and watches me
knees muddy, cup of tea growing cold:
and I rise up, no longer old nor the woman who waits
but grown strong from love songs
and long days spent in the sun,
and stronger still from all those days yet to come
for they could be the most precious yet.
So thank you for helping me to spend them well
it's something I will never forget.

1

Interprofessional ethics in everyday healthcare

Hilary Engward And Andrew Papanikitas

Introduction

Some form of interprofessional working (conceived broadly) is an every-day reality in healthcare across the globe. The premise underpinning care is that different professional groups can effectively work together to deliver good healthcare. This assumes that the communal activity of healthcare workers somehow adds up to better healthcare than that which is provided by one type of healthcare worker. Furthermore, interprofessional care has come to refer broadly both to conscious teamwork and the unconscious transition of healthcare work between individuals and teams (Clark et al., 2007; Wiles et al., 2016). This tends to present an ideal vision of people working together and knowing one another by name and role. However, this is not necessarily the case: doctors, nurses, physiotherapists, micro-biologists, radiologists, managers or lawyers might never meet, even if located in the same building, which often they are not. In addition to this, the interprofessional team may have differing employers, contracts, and professional agendas. The space where care decisions are made and enacted may be virtual – decisions (including those implicitly or explicitly ethical in nature) may be transacted online or via a telephone.

Accounts also suggest that interprofessional working does not always have a beneficial impact on patient care. Issues that compromise good interprofessional care include poor communication and a limited under-standing of others' roles and responsibilities. Such issues may manifest as interprofessional conflicts in patient care (Independent Police Complaints Commission, 2009). Whether or not these issues represent flawed examples of interprofessional working or ethical tensions inherent in them, their presence signals that there is scope for the useful study of interprofessional ethics.

Although there is much discussion about interprofessional working in the healthcare literature, there is relatively little work on the ethical issues that may be inherent in that working (whether it is working that is functional or working that is dysfunctional). This is ironic, firstly, because 'ethics' is a prominent feature in professional education for healthcare undergraduates; secondly, because most health professionals are likely to encounter care situations that fall outside their uni-professional expertise and remit, and will therefore call on the expertise of their fellow professions; and thirdly, that even if uni-professional knowledge and technical skills are not easily transferable across professions, ethics and values can be. This lack of looking into ethics in interprofessional working is perhaps a reason for a lack of meaningful discourse in interprofessional ethics education – it is because there is little insight into how ethics in interprofessional teams works. As such, education in interprofessional working tends to be 'dry' philosophy lectures to a diverse healthcare audience who are likely to find the content either irrelevant or simplistic. It is somewhat easier for diverse groups to want to sign up to a common, but perhaps superficially understood, set of values (Wiles et al., 2016) rather than a more challenging and nuanced approach.

The purpose of this chapter is therefore threefold: firstly, we clarify how we might better understand interprofessional working for the purpose of considering ethics at the interface between healthcare professions. Secondly, we consider the ethics of interprofessional working, and thirdly, what this might mean to making interprofessional education useful to the professions.

Clarifying 'interprofessional working'

Prior to exploring the ethical dimensions of interprofessional healthcare, the term *interprofessional* itself needs to be clarified. Leathard (2003) uses the term to refer to 'interactions between professionals involved, albeit from different backgrounds, but who have the same joint goals in working together'. This includes communication and decision-making, accountability, coordination, equality of resources, open communication, cooperation, assertiveness, autonomy, and mutual trust and respect. As such, interprofessional working is about team effectiveness, in which members of the team value one another's roles as important to the team's functionality.

The nature of teamwork and team performance in healthcare can be broadly categorised as favouring one of three types: multi-, inter- and trans-professional. 'Multi-' refers to different professions working each on their own goals in a rather autonomous way. 'Inter-' refers to them working closer together on a common goal and sharing a team identity, and 'trans-' refers to the disciplines or professions sharing competencies and therefore being able to take over tasks from other team members (Reeves et al., 2010). Inter- and trans-professional teamwork have been associated with enhanced team functioning and higher treatment quality (O'Leary et al., 2012); better clinical outcomes (Xyrichis and Lowton, 2008); improved patient safety (Salas et al., 2011); higher job satisfaction (Körner, 2010); and organisationally, increased cost savings and reduced turnover of staff (Zwarenstein et al., 2009). The implication in such categorisation is that some kinds of teamwork are better than others – the benefit which may be seen is both to service-users and to the healthcare workers themselves. Inter- and trans-professional healthcare have become the benchmarks of good teamwork in healthcare.

While effective teamwork may be an intrinsically valuable pursuit, it may also be that the prerequisites of effective team functionality bring about unique ethical challenges that are not necessarily seen in uni-professional settings. This is perhaps unsurprising as professions usually learn their basics in uni-professional settings, and although working with other professions may be addressed, it is still within the uni-professional classroom setting from that particular profession's perspective. For teams to function effectively, they are, however, required to have shared understandings about the purpose of each profession and an understanding as to how the individual works within a team. Understanding is insufficient, however, as team members must value and respect one another. This can be difficult if there is perceived hierarchy or if any members of the team are seen to be inferior or irrelevant by others in the same team (i.e. less worthy of respect or lacking in value). Any given healthcare worker may have a distinct set of goals, beliefs, values and physical demands associated with their profession, and often it is these distinctive features that are unobserved until they give rise to conflict – a phenomenon remarked upon by Fulford et al. in their work on values (Petrova et al., 2006). The everyday reality of the healthcare workplace may be that the individual works within a variety of teamwork structures, each with potential variety as to its function and as to how that team operates. Teamwork structures are ideally determined by the needs of patients, but also affected by political priorities and financial constraints. Teams will differ in their professional make-up and in their function to care for the patient (Papanikitas, 2008; Wiles et al., 2016). As such, ethics in interprofessional working needs to be more an ethics of teamwork rather than only ethics in inter- or trans-professional care.

To think about ethics of teamwork means we have to shift part of our focus away from the patient to include the team in our field of vision

(Clark et al., 2007). This does not mean that the patient ceases to be central to healthcare decision-making. Rather, in order for the patient to be best cared for, how teams work, and the ethics inherent in that working, need to be uncovered and unpacked. Indeed, it is in the needs of patients (and the failure to meet them) that we are likely to identify interprofessional issues that need to be aired. For example, as a young doctor, one of the authors commented on the risks posed to patient safety by the lack of effective communication between emergency obstetrics and emergency paediatrics. Each team, in the author's experience, had different priorities, different team structures and different processes (Papanikitas, 2008).

The purpose of ethics in relation to teamwork is firstly to acknowledge there are differences in how ethics is understood and used in the individual professions, and secondly how these ethics might talk to one another, with the potential that healthcare professionals can extend one another's moral gaze, rather than adopt a uniform vision that may be limiting for some team members.

Thinking about ethics in teamwork

Ethics is described in a great many ways in academia and education (Dowie and Martin, 2011). What makes it problematic in the interprofessional encounter is that it is perceived as the study of what is right or wrong, which includes the values and principles that govern individual, organisational and political conduct. As such, understanding ethics in interprofessional working needs to consider ethics as present in three differing, but interrelated, contexts – the individual encounter, the organisation within which that encounter occurs and the politics within which that practice is contained. It is important to note that no one context is more important than another. For example, if focus is primarily given to 'organisational shared values' or 'individual personal qualities', we risk ignoring the complicated interplay between people, policy, political ambitions and health outcomes – such phenomena that inform how people act and set limitations on possible courses of action and outcomes (Wintrup, 2015). The work of Clark et al. (2007) usefully complements this idea. They argue that how team members learn to negotiate with and understand one another depends upon three distinct but interrelated elements: (i) principles (guidelines for behaviour), (ii) structures (established forms of knowledge and patterns of behaviour) and (iii) processes (how things are done). We have chosen to adopt and build upon their framework here and elsewhere (Wiles et al., 2016; Engward, 2017).

Principles act as guidelines for behaviour

In healthcare, ethical issues are conceptualised in terms of codes of ethics (e.g. The Code: Professional Standards of Practice and Behaviour for Nurses and Midwives (NMC, 2015; Good Medical Practice [GMC], 2013). Most codes call for their professionals to work collaboratively with other professions (e.g. the NMC states that nurses/midwives must work cooperatively [clause 8] and share skills and knowledge for the benefit of patients and colleagues [clause 9]), and most practitioners would subscribe to this as being inherently a good thing. However, codes of ethics and standards themselves are usually developed with individual professions in mind and may be independent of context. The important point here is that different professions have different purposes. These different purposes may be a core element of what makes them that profession and may result in differences in priorities between different professionals in the interprofessional team. For example, the concept of confidentiality may have different emphasis between professions, leading to a nuanced application among, say, the GP, genito-urinary practitioner and social worker. For example, the general ethical focus (which includes the relative importance of confidentiality to other duties) may be on the individual and/or the family unit. Individual needs and family needs may differ and be difficult to navigate, where the issue of 'who' is being treated is relevant and may differ in relation to the purpose of the discipline in that team (for a worked example, see Wiles et al., 2016). As such, how confidentiality is understood and applied can differ across the professions because of the purpose of that profession. There is some support for the existence of such interprofessional ethical tensions; for example, Mitchelle (1982) found that nurses experience conflict in the interprofessional relationship due to different discourses in the professional–patient relationship, leading to a lack in coherence between what professionals feel they ought to do and what they actually do. Codes that are confined to such 'disciplinary silos' (Long et al., 2014) therefore risk uni-professional collegiality, in which professions pursue their own goals at the exclusion of other professions' goals (Hall, 2005).

Structures: established forms of knowledge and patterns of behaviour

A socio-historical perspective can be useful when considering how professions' socialisation nuances their interprofessional interactions with respect to ethics. Looking at the development of the professions, Freidson

(1988: pp xv) describes a profession as 'an occupation which has assumed a dominate position on a division of labour, so that it gains control over the determination of the substance of its own work'. How professions have historically evolved can indicate how professions worked together, which in turn informs how they currently work. For example, nursing was traditionally associated as a female occupation and viewed as less important than medicine, and as such, paid less, and this can be seen to filter into the clinical and practice context. Van der Lee et al. (2014) explored the historical development of the collaboration between obstetricians and midwives in Dutch maternity care. Findings showed that although both professions shared the same patient population and pursued the same goal, that is good maternity care, there was little interaction between the obstetricians and midwives, and what did exist was competitive rather than collaborative, where both professions used uni-professional protocols and strived to preserve autonomy in their professional practice. They found little evidence of interprofessional 'governance' and 'shared goals and vision'. Historically and culturally embedded perceptions about power between differing professions such as this are often implicit within practice, as opposed to being explicitly stated within governance and policy. They risk becoming part of a hidden curriculum.

This is not say that this occurs intentionally, but is rather unseen because it is not addressed. Where this is overtly expressed, then it may be the professions will learn and practice across one another. For example, Svantesson et al. (2008) explored whether interprofessional ethics rounds in nephrology units stimulated ethical reflection. The ethics rounds were associated with increased awareness of relations to other professions, including how other professionals think. Nurses gained an increased understanding of doctors, especially the doctors' 'loneliness' in trying to make the right decisions, and for some nurses, becoming more assertive in relation to the doctors' decision-making, such as questioning why dialysis treatment continued. The doctors, on the other hand, learned to understand other staff members' feelings of powerlessness and emotional connection to long-term patients. Besides new insights being directly connected to patients' situations, there was also insight that professionals shared the same view of the situation as difficult, as well as some reassurance that others have similar thoughts, thus reducing feelings of loneliness in decision-making; and others had their disciplinary pre-understandings confirmed, reinforcing how far doctors and nurses stand from each other.

These examples presented indicate that working, or collaborating, as a team is difficult, yet successful working requires some elements of collaboration. What becomes apparent is that different professions might interpret 'collaboration' differently. Holm et al. (1996) looked at ethics case discussions in mixed nurse-physician groups. They found that Danish physicians and nurses did not differ in the kind of ethical reasoning they use, but rather the physicians used more of the discussion time than nurses, used a more assertive style of argumentation, and the solutions chosen were usually first put forward by physicians. One implication of this commitment to teamwork arising from such insight is that doctors might interpret collaborate as 'lead' and nurses as 'facilitate', which in its turn could be a legacy of the socio-historical evolution of the medical and nursing professions.

Friend and Cook (1990) suggest that collaboration involves parity, mutual goals, shared accountability, shared resources and voluntariness. Here collaboration is neither top down nor bottom up, but rather acknowledges that each individual brings unique knowledge and skills that benefit the decision-making process. Although normative models of ethical thinking may be transferable across professions and practice contexts, how we talk about and make decisions about ethical dilemmas in diverse contexts needs to be discussed in order to be seen (something which has been referred to as a 'hermeneutic turn'). We previously mentioned that most professional learning occurs uni-professionally. In effect, we are not preparing professionals with the dialogic skills and language to be able to talk about ethics across the professions. As such, learning ethics of inter-professionalism, or teamwork, needs the skills to make sense of their ethics in relation to that particular team. This is difficult as it does not bring about immediate ethical resolution of a dilemma, which clinical practice often requires, but it may result in a resolution or change in a healthcare professional's original stance, perhaps leading toward richer interpretations and understandings of the multi-faceted natures of ethics and dilemma resolution.

Part of this new discourse about ethics of teams also requires the establishment of mutual goals. Mutuality is identified as the hallmark of collaboration, where goals must be acceptable to all involved. This entails some form of 'formalisation' and 'internalisation' of acceptable processes and limitations of practice, and although parity across the team is desired, it may be difficult to attain. In the van der Lee et al. study, formalisation of collaboration between the midwives and obstetricians entailed the introduction of regulations that tended to restrict midwifery practice to the physiological processes of pregnancy and delivery, without any usage of instruments or medication. This division may give obstetricians a dominant position over the midwives, but it also restricts the experience of midwives to physiological pregnancy and doctors to pathological pregnancy in ways that ultimately disadvantage patients.

Ethicists may have a role in acting as 'honest brokers' who see the different parts of the ethical puzzle and re-orientate the team to their shared goals. In one account of ethics rounds in a nephrology unite (Svantesson et al., 2008), a particular philosopher was admired for his ability to form structure and maintain discipline as well as balance the power between nurses and doctors. Many research and educational ethics forums that have been interdisciplinary comment on the value of shared interprofessional understanding of ethics in practice (Alderson et al., 2002). More academic attention needs to be focused, however, as to how such understandings have been informed or how things are being done while decisions are being made.

Processes – or how things are done

An understanding of the environment in which interprofessional ethics occurs is critical to developing a realistic approach. Where this is not taken into account we risk moral distress, the lingering distress that occurs when someone is prevented from fulfilling an ethical duty (Papanikitas, 2017). Understanding processes may enable conversations to occur about why some duties are not fulfilled – enabling individuals to understand where there is a moral duty to deviate from a local policy, and leaders to see when those policies need to change. Following we briefly discuss the importance of where and how things are done.

We have argued elsewhere that interprofessional teams in primary care may be geographically dispersed (King, 2007; Engward, 2017) and that interprofessional teams in hospital settings may have different perceived goals and responsibilities (Wiles et al., 2016). We would also argue, however, that geographical barriers can exist, albeit with smaller physical distance within institutions. As stated in the introduction, the members of the interprofessional team may never meet one another, may be geographically dispersed and may be subject to differing employment contracts, organisational agendas and professional regulation. The space where ethical decisions are made and enacted may be virtual or via a telephone, and members of the team may never meet one another. Due to such multivariate factors, healthcare professionals may experience difficulty in understanding each team member's role and responsibilities in the team, or how his or her role affects the patient's care. This can have a negative effect on a person's attitude towards collaboration and can inhibit collaboration skills (Van der Lee et al., 2013). For example, a study within the practices of UK general practitioners (GPs) showed that the extent of GPs' collaboration with, and patient referral to, allied health professionals was negatively influenced by the GPs' limited understanding of the roles and capabilities of those allied professionals (Baker et al., 2011).

A lack of understanding of one another's roles and responsibilities in the context of the wider healthcare system can lead to decision-making that pushes patients into the abandoned gaps between care. King (2007) uses a case study of a patient who requires wound dressing more often than the community can provide, and therefore has to access services at the local emergency department (ED). Simplistically viewed, the community team may have a moral duty, but not the resources. The ED team possibly have the resource (this too is debatable), but their primary duties are to a different population. Although changes in service provision and process may make internal sense, the patient is powerless to change or challenge the change, and may suffer harm as a result. Such an outcome is not necessarily an outcome of poor interprofessional teamwork or decision-making, but what it does demonstrate is that the patient is at the mercy of how the purposes of teams are set up, and the functions within those teams. In this case, there is a theoretical possibility that either team would not provide the dressing to a patient in need, but it does demonstrate that teams are working within resource-driven boundaries that do have a direct impact on the patient.

Conclusion

We have argued that it is important that interprofessional working, and the often invisible ethics inherent in that working, are better understood. The development of ethical discussion in relation to interprofessional teamwork fits with the direction of healthcare policy and practices in both Europe and other global settings. This includes better understanding the values and principles of conduct within which individuals practise. Applying a framework such as that used by Clark et al. (2007) enables us to see and explore different structures that influence interprofessional teamwork, centralising the wider principles, processes and structures the interprofessional team works within. In this context, for ethics to be its most useful, we need to ask questions about how care is able to be done within organisations and teams, and how teams become intrinsically ethical in their approach to their work. This is not to say that the individual is not important, but rather we suggest it is of equal importance to understand ethics as socio-culturally located in order to understand how interprofessional work ought to be. We refine Clark et al.'s model by suggesting that even intraprofessional (inter-speciality) accounts of ethical tension can and ought to be read as interprofessional accounts; for example, the 'obstetrician vs paediatrician' account (Papanikitas, 2008) is mentioned above because it is in fact a tension between emergency child health and emergency obstetric services and not, as the title suggests, a clash between any two individual doctors. We also suggest that the attention to processes may reveal that breaking down professional silos to create examples of interprofessional teamwork risks creating new silos. Whereas before there was a doctor silo and a nurse silo, there is now a child-health silo, a mental health silo, a maternity silo, within which gaps in service, and the ethics inherent within that service, can emerge.

Some form of interprofessional working (conceived broadly) is an everyday reality in healthcare across the globe, even if it does not aim to be inter- or transdisciplinary (conceived narrowly). As such, for a more nuanced understanding of ethics in interprofessional working, some translational work is needed. By this we mean a better empirically based understanding is needed to explore working realities of interprofessional healthcare, but we also need to re-explore what we already know of healthcare ethics in relation to contexts of healthcare. We have demonstrated in the above chapter that the interprofessional space has the potential to be ethically problematic, and that implies risk to patient safety and healthcare quality. Further work is needed – theoretical and empirical that will connect academia, education and practice if this ethical risk is to be addressed.

References

Alderson, P., Farsides, B. and Williams, C. (2002) Examining ethics in practice: health service professionals' evaluations of in-hospital ethics seminars. *Nurse Ethics*, 9(5), pp. 8–21.

Baker, L., Egan-Lee, E., Martimianakis, M.A., et al. (2011) Relationships of power: implications for inter-professional education. *Journal of Inter-professional Care*, 25, pp. 98–104.

Braunack-Mayer, A. (2007) The ethics of primary health care, in R. Ashcroft, H. Draper, A. Dawson and J. McMillan (eds), *Principles of Healthcare Ethics* (pp. 357–64). 2nd edn. London: Wiley.

Clark, P., Cott, C. and Drinka, T. (2007) Theory and practice in inter-professional ethics: a framework for understanding ethical issues in healthcare teams. *Journal of Inter-professional Care*, 21(6), pp. 591–603.

De Vries, R.G. (2004) *A Pleasing Birth: Midwives and Maternity Care in the Netherlands*. Philadelphia, PA: Temple University Press.

Dowie, A. and Martin, A. (2011) Clarifying ethics and law in the curriculum. *Ethics and Law in the Medical Curriculum*. Dundee: Association for Medical Education in Europe.

Engward, H. (2017) Inter-professional ethics in the primary care setting. Chapter 3, in A. Papanikitas and J. Spicer (eds), *Handbook of Primary Care Ethics* (pp. 197–202). Abingdon, UK: CRC Press.

Freidson, E. (1988) *Profession of Medicine: A study of the sociology of applied knowledge,* Chicago: The university of chicago press.

Friend, M. and Cook, K. (1990) Collaboration as a prediction for success in school reform. *Journal of Educational Psychological Consultation,* 1, pp. 69–86.

Hall, P. (2005) Inter-professional teamwork: professional cultures as barriers. *Journal of Inter-professional Care,* 19, pp. 188–96.

General Medical Council (2013) *Good Medical Practice.* General Medical Council.

Holm, S., Gjersoe, P., Grode, G., Hartling, O., Ibsen, K.E. and Marcussen, H. (1996) Ethical Reasoning in mixed nurse-physician groups. *Journal of Medical Ethics,* 22:168–73.

Independent Police Complaints Commission (2009) Report into contact between Fiona Pilkington and Leicester constabulary 2004–2007. https://www.ipcc.gov.uk/investigations/fiona-pilkington-leicestershire-police.

King, A. (2007) Inter-professional team working: a moral endeavour? An exploration of clinical practice using Seedhouse's ethical grid, in D. Bowman and J. Spicer (eds), *Primary Care Ethics* (pp. 100–15). Abingdon: Radcliffe Publishing.

Körner, M. (2010) Inter-professional teamwork in medical rehabilitation: a comparison of multidisciplinary and interdisciplinary team approach. *Clinical Rehabilitation,* 24, pp. 745–55.

Leathard, A. (2003) The meaning of the words, in Leathard, A. (ed.), *Inter-professional Collaboration: From Policy to Practice in Health and Social Care* (pp. 5–6). London: Routledge.

Long, T., Dann, S., Wolff, M.L. and Brienze, R.S. (2014) Moving from silos to teamwork: integration of inter-professional trainees into a medical home model. *Journal of Inter-professional Care,* 28, pp. 473–74.

Mitchelle, C. (1982) Integrity in inter-professional relationships. In: Agich G.J. (eds) *Responsibility in Health Care.* Philosophy and Medicine, vol 12. Springer, Dordrecht pp. 163–84 https://link.springer.com/chapter/10.1007/978-94-009-7831-7_9#citeas.

NMC (2015) *The Code: Professional Standards of Practice and Behaviour for Nurses and Midwives.* London: Nursing and Midwifery Council.

O'Leary, K.J., Sehgal, N.L., Terrell, G. and Williams, M.V. (2012) Interdisciplinary teamwork in hospitals: a review and practical recommendations for improvement. *Journal of Hospital Medicine,* 7, pp. 48–54.

Papanikitas, A.N. (2008) Obstetrician vs. paediatrician: does inter-professional indifference compromise emergency caesarean safety? *International Journal of Surgery* (London, England), 6(1), pp. 5–6.

Papanikitas, A. (2017) Self-awareness and professionalism. *InnovAiT,* 10, pp. 452–57.

Pellegrino, E. (1983) The healing relationship: the architronics of clinical medicine, in Shelp, E.A. (ed.), *The Clinical Encounters: The Moral Fabric of the Patient-Physician Relationship* (p. 679). Dordrecht: Reidel Publishing Company.

Petrova, M., Dale, J. and Fulford, B.K. (2006) Values-based practice in primary care: easing the tensions between individual values, ethical principles and best evidence. *British Journal of General Practice*, 56, pp. 703–9.

Reeves, S., Lewin, S., Espin, S. and Zwarenstein, M. (2010) *Inter-professional Teamwork for Health and Social Care*. Chichester: West Sussex: Blackwell.

Salas, E., Gregory, M.E. and King, H.B. (2011) Team training can enhance patient safety–the data, the challenge ahead. *Joint Commission Journal on Quality and Patient Safety/Joint Commission Resources*, 37, pp. 339–40.

Svantesson, M., Anderzén-Carlsson, A., Thorsén, H., Kallenberg, K. and Ahlström, G. (2008) Inter-professional ethics rounds concerning dialysis patients: staff's ethical reflections before and after rounds. *Journal of Medical Ethics*, 34(5), pp. 407–13.

Van der Lee, N., Driessen, E.W., Houwaart, E.S., Caccia, N.C. and Scheele, F. (2014) An examination of the historical context of inter-professional collaboration in Dutch obstetrical care. *Journal of Inter-professional Care*, 28, pp. 123–27.

Van der Lee, N., Fokkema, J.P., Westerman, M., Driessen, E.W., van der Vleuten, C.P., Scherpbier, A.J.J.A. and Scheele, F. (2013) The CanMEDS framework: relevant but not quite the whole story. *Medical Teacher*, 35, pp. 949–55.

Wiles K., Bahal N., Engward, H. and Papanikitas, A. (2016) Ethics in the interface between multidisciplinary teams: a narrative in stages for inter-professional education. *London Journal of Primary Care*, 8(6), pp. 100–4, DOI: 10.1080/17571472.2016.1244892.

Wintrup, J. (2015) The changing landscape of care: does ethics education have a new role to play in health practice. *BMC Medical Ethics*, 16, p. 22.

Xyrichis, A. and Lowton, K. (2008) What fosters or prevents inter-professional teamworking in primary and community care? A literature review. *International Journal of Nursing Studies*, 45, pp. 140–53.

Zwarenstein, M., Goldman, J. and Reeves, S. (2009) Inter-professional collaboration: effects of practice-based interventions on professional practice and healthcare outcomes. Cochrane Database of Systematic Reviews, Jul 8;(3):CD000072, DOI: 10.1002/14651858.CD000072.pub2.

2

An ethics of care transformation of mental health service provision: creating services that people want to use

Tula Brannelly

Introduction

People who use mental health services are continually subjected to a lack of the basic human and civil rights available to other citizens (Drew et al., 2011), including fundamental freedoms such as the right to liberty and to refuse medical interventions. These actions are (contentiously) justified, even mandated, to prevent serious harm, such as in life-threatening situations. However, most compulsion is not used in this way. Newer legislation in the UK, such as community treatment orders (CTOs), has extended controls into various aspects of life requiring people to take medications, attend clinician appointments, decide where the person must live or attend vocational schemes (Rugkasa and Burns, 2009), often long term.

Where inpatient detention is used, there is the issue of reported increasing levels of violence on non-forensic wards in 'high-income countries' (Iozzino et al., 2015). Although this suggests that the use of force and detention produces its own culture of relation between the users and providers of services, most research focuses on the psychiatric and addiction categorisations of those identified as high risk, such as males, those with a schizophrenic type illness or a secondary alcohol use disorder (see, for example, Iozzino et al., 2015). Although psychiatric categorisations, gender and risk have been heavily critiqued, increasingly attention is given to the abuse and violence experienced through the relationships between service users and mental health workers from the perspective of mental health service users who have been detained.

Commonly, it is thought that mental health legislation is used either to protect 'the public' from people who may be dangerous or to protect people from themselves. Less visible are the details of the circumstances in which detention and compulsory treatment are used, whether they are a proportionate response to a person's distress, or that protection is what is needed and valued by the service user. This raises important questions about how services are experienced, and therefore whether they are effective in providing the care that people need. If the aim of service provision is protection, then whom are services aiming to protect? Is protection what the person using services needs? What constitutes the need for protection? Is the care provided adequate for the level of distress the person is experiencing? Is the care provided able to help people make sense of the distress they are experiencing? What works for the person in distress to reduce the need for protection?

Mental health workers have a key role in assessment and treatment of people with mental health problems, and they contribute to the enforcement of legislation. Legislative processes have an impact on the therapeutic relationship, and people who use services are clear that the relationship cannot be therapeutic given the power imbalance. The use of force has been described by people who have experience of services as the 'boulder in the road' to achieving recovery-focused services (Brannelly, 2015). Experiences of coercion are reported (Owen and Floyd, 2010), and interventions such as seclusion and restraint are sites of (re)traumatisation, prompting targeted decreases in their use. Meanwhile, there is little conceptualisation or critique of what is, or is not, care in mental healthcare provision.

In this article, the ethics of care (Tronto, 1993, 2013) is used as a framework to surface what is care, what is protection and what is not care in mental health service provision. Integral to this approach is the broader aim of challenging the marginalisation and subjugation of certain groups by asking whether current practices are just. This paper considers care ethics and mental health by surfacing some of the current discussions and contradictions that impact on the experiences of people who have a mental health problem, drawing on a small qualitative research study with mental health service user activists in England and Aotearoa New Zealand.[1]

[1] Acknowledgement: I would like to thank the service users who have influenced my research and education over the years, particularly *Suresearch* in Birmingham, *Te Waka Whaiora* and the *Wellink Youth Governance Group* in Wellington as well as others who have added fuel to the fire of renewal. This research was not funded.

Methodology

This small qualitative research project, entitled 'Acts of Citizenship' (after Isin and Nielson, 2008), examined priorities for change in mental health service provision. Working alongside mental health service users in research and education inevitably included conversations about what could be different in service provision. I decided to do this research project to explore service change priorities from the perspectives of people active in service user movements. The research participants were service user activists (they may not refer to themselves as such) from Aotearoa New Zealand (6) and England (3); seven women and two men. Participants often had long-standing careers as advocates, commissioners and commentators. Initially, three participants were approached who were known to be active in governance and advocacy roles, and they suggested others that may participate. In addition, one service user group in England was approached to advertise the project, and three participants were contacted via this group. Seven interviews were face to face; one by telephone and one participant responded by email. The participants were asked to comment on key aspects of citizenship for people who use services and current priorities for change identified by service user organisations that they were part of, for them personally. Ethics agreement was gained through Massey University Human Ethics Committee in New Zealand.

The data were analysed using the stages of thematic analysis (Braun and Clarke, 2006). Unequivocally, when asked what the priorities were for change in mental health services, the use of force, compulsory treatment and detention were foremost and raised questions about the experiences of compulsion. The experience of compulsion was experienced as a lack of care. Any outcome that was achieved through the intervention could have been done so in a way that did not include the use of compulsion. This contrasted sharply with the policy priorities of improved access, increased variety of services and decreased waiting times. In the next section, data relating to compulsion are presented, followed by a discussion of Tronto's three moral boundaries to shed light on these experiences and consider the transformations required to existing service provision.

Experiences of compulsion and reflections on governance roles

In this research, compulsion was rarely discussed as an aid to recovery. More frequently, the mental health legislation was viewed as an unnecessarily heavy and unconstructive response to distress, a way of guaranteeing access to inpatient services at a time of severe resource constraint or a way of extending continuing controls.

> So that, compulsory treatment has got to be the hot issue – that is the issue that is stopping services developing, it is the boulder in the middle of the road to achieve a recovery-orientated service ... One of the conflations that happens in this debate is that people associate compulsory treatment with reliable services. So they think if we didn't have that there, my relative would be neglected. (Lizzie)

One participant reflected on her role as a mental health commissioner who advocated for people in long-term detention.

> Although I have worked as a Mental Health Act Commissioner for a long time, I still cannot see the rationale for a lot of the people that I visit that are detained that they are still detained, even if it had been right that they were in an initial position where they had to be taken from their home or something. Even then, I don't think there is any justification for it ... Compulsion ruins everything. (Teresa)

Participants described their experiences – surprise at being placed under mental health legislation, not knowing the criteria for assessment, compulsion or discharge. One participant noted that the assessment of risk that prompted the use of the act was seldom understood. While a voluntary patient, she described wanting to pop home to check that someone was looking after her cat.

> The ward was not locked and I wanted to get home to check on my cat and I walked out and walked straight into my psychiatrist walking the other way. And he said, right ICU [intensive care unit] with you and suddenly I had five nurses on top of me dragging me to ICU. I got put under the Act. So, I just wanted to leave and no one said to me well why do you want to leave and I can come with you to check on your cat, if they had done I would have been fine. (Katie)

Another participant discussed how, when the Act was used, staff adopted an assumption of total loss of contact with reality, or a complete loss of competence. A staff member was surprised that someone under the Act was able to respond appropriately when moved to an emergency department, for example.

> I had an experience, kind of like a tachycardia while in [inpatient ward] and my pulse rate was so high, I thought my body was going to explode and they were very poorly able to respond to the physicality of what was happening,

and so I was put in the ambulance and taken to the general hospital in [city]. And I had a young nurse that came with me, and we went through the ED [emergency department] process, and every stage she kept saying 'oh my god you're the most sane person here'. But I was 'specialled' she had to be with me the whole time ... she said you're making the sanest appraisal of what's going on here, she was completely blown away by the fact that here I was stuck under a Mental Health Act, able to see in some way and make some sort of sense of what was happening in a very busy ED situation. Because I was the one that was under the Act, and therefore had some kind of chaotic inability to perceive reality. (Josephine)

Another area of concern was compulsory treatment, especially with medications that were harmful. The participants discussed the use of quick-acting medications such as Accuphase administered at times when the person needed time to come to grips with his or her situation, rather than drug-induced confusion and sedation. But of more concern were medications that are taken long term, that have harmful side effects, such as dramatic weight gain resulting in Type 2 diabetes and heart disease.

It's actually tragic. And the drugs that are sanctioned are life-shortening, and not only that some people are forced to take them indefinitely, it is not even a choice and I find it outrageous and no one seems to be concerned about it. (Lizzie)

Despite a long-term policy aim of the reduction in the use of seclusion, the participants noted that in meetings, for example with senior mental health service managers, seclusion and restraint were discussed as unquestionably necessary. Where new wards were designed, even with service user participation, they featured seclusion areas.

One of the strong issues for consumers has for a long time been involuntary treatment, particularly seclusion and the use of force, and I saw that he, the director general, in spite of the ministry having a policy apparently of eventual elimination of seclusion [in New Zealand], well he himself said he believed there would always be a need for seclusion, he said that at a minuted meeting, so when you've got that's the view of the chief psychiatrist, that's very hard. (Martin)

The participants discussed how people commonly thought that interventions such as the use of seclusion were historical, located sometime in the past, and were met with surprise when they explained that the use of seclusion continued today. Two participants wondered what we would think looking back at this era of mental health service provision and its brutality felt by those using services, and thought that we, as a global society, would have wanted to act more dramatically to make change.

> I don't know if in my lifetime we'll see seclusion eliminated but it's like that to me is one of the kind of, it's a hallmark from an era that in itself if it was accomplished, would signify a great movement towards recognising that, and distress or kind of mind chaos, however you want to frame the experience, people need things; that they do not need to be shut off from other human beings. It just seems so simple to me. (Josephine)

One participant reflected on her experiences of seclusion over decades of mental health service use. It was experienced as brutality, and she talked of other kinds of intervention that are available.

> I read about a woman's experience that seemed so similar. A group took her and looked after her and fed her, and she wasn't shut away from that which was so familiar to her was nurtured, she wasn't asked to explain herself and she kind of came out the other end of this profound understanding of what she learnt, and in a state of healthiness that I thought, stunning, and that little story has stayed with me most of my life because the responses I've had have always been far from that: shut off, injected, get back out there, try and create a life for yourself; and it seems so brutal. (Josephine)

This small group of participants offered alternatives to what was available, and described some current practices that should be immediately removed to improve the situation for people who use services. The alternatives sit within a service user–focused recovery framework (not a co-option of the recovery framework), and the practices included the removal of any treatment without consent and the recognition of the experience of (re)traumatisation because of the use of physical force. In the next section of this paper, I move on to discuss the implications of these ideas, framed using the ethics of care.

Tronto's moral boundaries

The ethics of care (Tronto, 1993) questions the moral boundaries that sustain prevalent structural and intersectional inequalities. Tronto (1993, pp. 6–10) contested three moral boundaries: morality and politics, the moral 'point of view', and public and private life. Morality and politics are entirely entwined, and Tronto argues that care can serve as the moral value and political achievement of a good society.

Moral boundary 1 – morality and politics

In relation to achieving justice for people who experience mental health problems, care as a value and a political achievement questions the morality and the political action that sustain oppression and marginalisation for some groups of people. Asking these questions surfaces a conversation that is currently framed very differently in terms of rights and professional expertise.

A call for social justice is made when a particular group is acknowledged as consistently marginalised. One condition for a free society is to consider inequalities associated with marginalised groups, and therefore that freedom is measured not in the level of choice that a person has in a neoliberal sense of self-determination, but in the attention paid to the pursuit of equality (Tronto, 2013). Another condition is to question protectionism both to and for citizens, such as toward some citizens within society, marginalised by their citizenship status, and toward others seen as a threat to citizenship. As currently stands, people who experience mental health problems have an added jeopardy of the potential for state-sanctioned actions toward them to hinder their recovery. In the UK, benefit sanctions and housing crises are two examples affecting the well-being of people with mental health problems. So access to adequate housing may be difficult, but the drugs that are not wanted will be forced upon them.

Overall, people who are marginalised are more likely to develop long-term mental health problems alongside multiple structural discriminations (Graham, 2009). People who have enduring mental health problems are more likely to experience poverty, long-term unemployment and poor employment opportunities. People with major psychiatric diagnoses, such as schizophrenia and depression, are likely to die younger (Craig, 2008). The New Zealand Mental Health Commission found that 80 per cent of people with long-term mental health problems are unemployed – the highest of any group with disabilities (Mental Health Commission, 2011). Stigma and discrimination within communities and families is common (Barnett and Barnes, 2010), as is self-stigma (Peterson, 2007). The relationship between deprivation or childhood adversity and significant mental health problems in later life is often understated but should not be dismissed (Bentall et al., 2014), as trauma is emerging as a direct influence in voice hearing and other long-term conditions.

Indigenous communities may be retraumatised by the colonial implications of mental health assessment and treatment, particularly where services are unable to connect people with indigenous healers. Experiences that are culturally valued may be dismissed as mental illness. In Aotearoa New Zealand, the indigenous Māori population and Pacific

Island people are overrepresented in mental health services (Oakley-Browne et al., 2006), particularly in terms of compulsory treatment and detention. Little is known about how some different cultural groups understand mental health and illness, such as Tongans in Aotearoa, New Zealand (Vaka et al., 2016).

People who access services experience very poor outcomes, while mental health services are under increasing pressure. A community survey in New Zealand suggests that 20 per cent of the population have a level of distress that constitutes a diagnosable mental illness at any time, with half of the population likely to experience distress of these levels across their lifespan (Oakley et al., 2006). According to the UK charity Mind, one in four people will experience a mental health problem at any time. Mental illness is, in fact, so common that it is possible to question whether it is 'abnormal' as defined by psychiatric classification (nikolasrose.com). Despite its common occurrence, access to effective help is not readily available, for example in primary care, where disclosure is deterred by the fear of the consequences (Dew et al., 2007).

A current trend holds that mental health should be taken seriously, for example in England, where it has been identified as a priority for change. The current situation must be addressed. Positioning people with mental health problems as abnormal, offering unavailable or stigmatising services with ineffective or iatrogenic treatments, responses that reinforce loss and increase the risk of multiple inequalities, indicates that an alternative view is overdue. As the quotes above demonstrate, obstacles to being heard and responded to result in trauma to people who use services that is unnecessary and unhelpful.

Moral Boundary 2 – the moral point of view

The philosophical position of morality sees it as distanced and objective. But in the ethics of care, a distant and disinterested position is not one from which to make moral observations. Placing morality in a realm of reason without emotional connection makes it universal rather than situated, and hierarchical and focused on the content of moral thought rather than action orientated. The moral point of view in relation to mental health often refers to the eminence of autonomy, which champions reason, agency and logic. The problem this presents is that this particular moral point of view translates as a clinical indicator of mental illness where people are judged on 'insight', judgement and capacity; often deemed lacking abilities in these areas; and therefore unable to have any control in their own lives. This negates usual decision-making processes which include the person's social network. It demeans the experience of distress where reason, agency and logic may be acquiescent to understanding more personal and interpersonal dynamics and causes of distress.

Approaching people with an open or closed response has very different implications for what can be constituted in the relationship, and the opportunities for that relationship. An open response is one that recognises and acknowledges the other, and is an epistemological approach to care (Barnes, 2012). A closed response is where the other is silenced through the action of interpretation, presented as knowledge, and is a response that results in epistemological violence (Teo, 2010) where experience is dismissed as invalid through psychiatric classification and interpretation. The clinical assessment interview and other clinical interactions are prime sites for the possibility of open or closed responses. One aspect of the clinical interview is the requirement for mental health workers to translate the experience of the person in distress into clinical language through clinical interpretation using a diagnostic classification system; even the most sensitive of practitioners struggle to maintain the essence of the experience as part of the translation into clinical terminology. A possible result of the translation is a homogenisation of experience whereby the meaning associated with the experience is lost and that experiences are grouped into activities demarcated as 'risky' or 'non-risky'.

Recent developments in the ethics of care have recentralised the connection between care ethics, politics and justice (Tronto, 2013; Barnes, 2012; Barnes et al., 2015). In relation to mental health, this has to raise the question about why certain people who have certain experiences, categorised in certain ways, are positioned to lose their citizenship. The voices of mental health service users are absolutely key in understanding how to restore justice and citizenship. Only people who experience service use have the perspective on whether the service met their needs.

Moral Boundary 3 – public and private life

Tronto's third moral boundary is the boundary between public and private life. Recently, I spent some time assessing a staff member on an 'acute care' area of an in-patient psychiatric unit, a small locked area with five rooms used for seclusion, adjacent to, but separate from, the larger inpatient unit. The five small locked rooms were all occupied, and two nurses sat in a smaller room with a transparent plastic screen. Access to basic facilities was very limited, and privacy was not an option. The environment was very poor, and it was difficult to see how such an environment is conducive to practices of care and recovery, one that enables staff and people who use services to work in a way that promotes health and well-being.

The private world of mental health service provision is not visible or known to people outside of it, but is experienced as traumatic by many who are subjected to it. Care ethics suggests that to achieve the good society, people have a moral responsibility to one another (Tronto, 1993; Sevenhuijsen, 1998), and people with privilege are in a position that enables the mobilisation of political will and action to make change that ameliorates rather than sustains social inequalities (Young, 2006). Inertia represents what Tronto (2009) and Barnes (2012) referred to as 'privileged irresponsibility', where the main benefactors of care do not register its value. Care is pivotal to taking responsibility, and taking responsibility is pivotal to action (Walker, 2007).

People require knowledge to act, and therefore actions are reproductions of pre-existing structures, so those structures may be reproduced (Giddens, 1984). Similarly, Bourdieu (1980, as cited in Young, 2006) sees actions as limited by the possibilities for interpretation that each offers the other. Lévinas (1998) suggests that openness to the other or interpretation of the other are momentary choices made within the relationship – to be able to understand the other as distinct and different in the social relation or to interpret the other according to what is already known. In an attempt to surface hidden practices, to inform the political through the personal, it is essential to understand the experiences of people subject to such actions, as sought through this small research project.

Care or protection?

In this context of mental health service provision, the separation of care and protection as two distinctly different activities has two benefits. Firstly, the actions required for protection may be care. Secondly, if circumstances arise where protection is required, once the cause of the need for protection has dissipated, protection is no longer required. Users of mental health services recognise over-involvement of services as a control of behaviours rather than a clinical intervention to help a person into recovery and out of crisis (Slade et al., 2012). 'Personal recovery' regards ongoing clinical service intervention as antithetical to recovery, precisely because long-term involvement does not enable people to access other means of recovery and ties people into a system that is focused more on identification of problems and clinical interventions that ask people to self-survey for symptoms. A constant state of alertness to an onset of symptoms does not provide the kind of atmosphere where people can find the space to recover (Scott and Wilson, 2011).

The overprotective approach adopted by many of the world's mental health services is based on constructions of providing safety and avoiding risk. Tronto (1993, p. 105) recognises that protection can become 'self-serving' as a 'protection racket'. In this protection racket, protection is propagated by the actions of those who protect, removing focus from people who require control. Protection is different to caring; it creates a different relationship. It assumes a threat or intention of harm from the individual to the group, and a response to that threat (Tronto, 1993, p. 105). This raises a number of issues. The first is the purpose of detention and forced treatment and what it is hoped they will achieve. If the aim is to protect, then to intervene is just, and this is care as long as it is experienced as such. Recovery-orientated services suggest that to have to resort to detention or forced treatment is an indication of a failure of service intervention and should be the starting point for the implementation of recovery (Gordon, 2013).

The second is what treatment is on offer. Often this is the use of antipsychotic medications that may have limited efficacy, but many side effects, such as dramatic weight gain, that put people off taking them for good reason. Although there is little evidence concerning the criteria for the use of protection, it is not only in the circumstances of life-threatening conditions that mental health legislation is implemented and used for many years of people's lives. For a small number of citizens, being under the Act is constant surveillance and adherence by mental health services, often without the ability to meaningfully intervene in people's lives in a positive way to improve living standards or conditions. As people in this situation are likely to have already experienced a lifetime of trauma and perhaps abuse or addiction, increasing the levels of attention needed to ameliorate the impact of these on daily life is what is required, rather than the response that is available currently.

Conclusion

If we attend to people who use services as a group of people who are marginalised, based on the knowledge that they fare worse than other citizens, then it is just to consider what may change to promote equality. The ethics of care guides this thinking. The first is the question of equality, and here it is possible to highlight the issues of concern that demarcate mental health service users as an unequal group. The second is to use Tronto's integrity of care to both guide and critique care practices.

The first aspect requires the political focus that Tronto's work affords – identification of structural discriminations, questioning the positioning of certain groups that results from the values and norms of society and how people are constructed into subject positions, and how resources are allocated for care. Over recent years, mental health legislation has extended its reach. When the use of community-based legislation was proposed in the 2007 review of the Mental Health Act in England, there was considerable concern from professionals about how these controls could be practised, the types of treatments on offer and the impacts on recovery for people subject to them. The critique of the widening encapsulation of abnormality through the psychiatric cataloguing of behaviours through technologies such as the Diagnostic Statistics Manual also provides a challenge. Services have to engage with their shortcomings for meeting the needs of the community (Mezzina et al., 2006). Neoliberalist ideals of the productive, consuming and rational citizen are also unhelpful for people who find themselves pathologised and excluded, locating illness and dependence with the citizen while ignoring discriminatory practices within society.

Service user and survivor movements have sought to establish a centrality of voice for people who use services. Inclusion of service users in governance at many levels has been hailed as the most promising leverage for change and transformation of service provision, and yet that transformation remains to be seen. As Barnes (2012) points out, putting people in a room together does not result in a change in the power dynamic or a meaningful acceptance of responsibility for change. Yet it is precisely this process that is required in order to connect together those who have power and those who know what needs to change, in order to take responsibility for transformation.

Mary O'Hagan, in her book *Madness Made Me* (2013), outlined the lack of interest in her as a person and the low expectations that services had about her life in ways that are familiar to professionals who have been involved in services for some time. Things have changed. No longer are people routinely told that they are not expected to be a person who contributes to society through work and family; but in more subtle ways people continue to be discouraged. Citizenship in mental health is about belonging to communities, legal status as a relationship with the state and about the positioning and value given to some humans. It is complex, interweaved, influential and evident in the kinds of responses that people experience. That discrimination continues to the extent and degree that it does needs to be recognised and challenged, and that communities continue to ostracise people with mental illness needs attention. The relationship between the state and individuals is operationalised through the practices of paid workers, who would also like to work within a system that enables them to provide the sort of help that is needed. Given these arguments for the transformation of services, their continuation without transformation is intriguing.

I became aware of the ethics of care as a PhD student researching rights for people with dementia, and immediately thought that it could have been useful to guide complex practice decisions as a (previous mental health) practitioner. But it is also broader than practice and allows critique and interrogation of the political and philosophical values and concepts that underpin practice, policy and research. Beyond critique and interrogation, it also enables renewal, and this may lead us into a more enlightened future of mental health service provision. What we have at the moment is not working for our communities. Waiting times are too long to get specialist services; people with experience are not readily available to people in distress; responses that lack humanity such as seclusion are commonplace; and some medications that are prescribed are harmful. In this critical moment, transformation and renewal are required, and an ethics of care is a way of thinking about the world that can allow that to happen.

References

Barnes, M. (2012) *Care in Everyday Life*. Bristol: Policy Press.

Barnes, M., Brannelly, T., Ward, L. and Ward, N. (2015) *Ethics of Care – Critical Advances in International Perspective*. Bristol: Policy Press.

Barnett, H. and Barnes, A. (2010). *Walk a Mile in Our Shoes/He tuara, ngā tapuwae tuku iho ō ngā Mātua Tūpuna: Exploring Discrimination Within and Towards Families and Whānau of People Diagnosed with 'Mental Illness'*. Auckland: Mental Health Foundation of New Zealand.

Bentall, R.P., de Sousa, P., Varese, F., Wickham, S., Sitko, K., Haarmans, M. and Read J. (2014) From adversity to psychosis: pathways and mechanisms from specific adversities to specific symptoms. *Social Psychiatry Psychiatric Epidemiology*, 49, pp. 1011–22, DOI: 10.1007/s00127-014-0914-0.

Brannelly, T. (2015) Mental health service use and the ethics of care: in pursuit of justice. In M. Barnes, T. Brannelly, L. Ward and N. Ward (eds), *Ethics of Care – Critical Advances in International Perspectives*. Bristol: Policy Press.

Braun, V. and Clarke, V. (2006) Using thematic analysis in psychology. *Qualitative Research in Psychology*, 3(2), pp. 77–101, DOI: 10.1191/1478088706qp063oa.

Craig, T.J. (2008) Major psychiatric disorders increase risk of mortality. *Evidence-Based Mental Health*, 11, p. 9, DOI: 10.1136/ebmh.11.1.9.

Dew, K., Morgan, S., Dowell, A., McLoed, D., Bushnell, J. and Collings, S. (2007) It puts things out of your control: fear of consequences as a barrier to patient disclosure of mental health issues to general practitioners. *Sociology of Health and Illness*, 29(7), pp. 1059–74, DOI: 10.1111/j.1467-9566.2007.01022.x.

Drew, N., Funk, M., Tang, S. et al. (2011) Human rights violations of people with mental and psychosocial disabilities: an unresolved global crisis. *The Lancet*, 378, pp. 1664–75, DOI: 10.1016/S0140-6736(11)61458-X.

Gordon, S. (2013) The recovery of compulsory assessment and treatment'. In J. Dawson and K. Gledhill (eds), *New Zealand's Mental Health Act in Practice*. Wellington: Victoria University Press.

Graham, H. (2009) *Understanding Health Inequalities*. Maidenhead: Open University Press.

Giddens, A. (1984) *The Constitution of Society: Outline on the Theory of Structuration*. California: University of California Press.

Iozzino, L., Ferrari, C., Large, M., Nielssen, O. and de Girolamo, G. (2015) Prevalence and risk factors of violence by psychiatric acute inpatients: a systematic review and meta-analysis. *PLoS ONE*, 10(6), p. e0128536, DOI: 10.1371/journal.pone.0128536.

Isin, E.F. and Nielson, G.M. (2008) *Acts of Citizenship*. Chicago, IL: University of Chicago Press.

Lévinas, E. (1998) *On Thinking-of-the-Other: Entre Nous*, trans. Smith, M.B. and Harshav, B. New York: Columbia University Press.

Mental Health Commission. (2011) *Measuring Social Inclusion, People with Experience of Mental Distress and Addiction*. Wellington: Mental Health Commission.

Mezzina, R., Davidson, L., Borg, M., Marin, I., Topor, A. and Sells, D. (2006) The social nature of recovery: discussion and implications for practice. *American Journal of Psychiatric Rehabilitation*, 9(1), pp. 63–80, DOI: 10.1080/1548776 0500339436.

O'Hagan, M. (2014) *Madness Made Me*. Wellington: Open Box.

Oakley Browne, M.A., Wells, J.E. and Scott, K.M. (eds). (2006) *Te Rau Hinengaro The New Zealand Mental Health Survey*. Wellington: Ministry of Health.

Owen, J.L. and Floyd, M. (2010) Negotiated coercion: thoughts about involuntary treatment in mental health. *Ethics and Social Welfare*, 4(3), pp. 297–99.

Peterson, D. (2007) *I Haven't Told Them, They Haven't Asked*. Auckland: Mental Health Foundation of New Zealand.

Rugkasa, J. and Burns, T. (2009) Community treatment orders. *Psychiatry*, 8(12), pp. 493–95.

Scott, A. and Wilson, L. (2011) Valued identities and deficit identities: wellness recovery action planning and self-management in mental health. *Nursing Inquiry*, 18 (1): 40–49, DOI: 10.1111/j.1440-1800.2011.00529.x.

Sevenhuijsen, S. (1998) *Citizenship and the Ethics of Care: Feminist Considerations on Justice, Morality and Politics*. London: Routledge.

Slade, M., Adams, N. and O'Hagan, M. (2012) Editorial, recovery: past progress and future challenges. *International Review of Psychiatry*, February 2012, 24(1), pp. 1–4, DOI: 10.3109/09540261.2011.644847.

Teo, T. (2010) What is epistemological violence in the empirical social sciences? *Social and Personality Psychology Compass*, 4(5), pp. 295–303, DOI: 10.1111/j.1751-9004.2010.00265.x.

Tronto, J.C. (1993) *Moral Boundaries – A Political Argument for an Ethic of Care*. London: Routledge.

Tronto, J.C. (2009) Consent as a grant of authority: a care ethics reading of informed consent. In H. Lindeman, M. Verkerk and M.U. Walker (eds),

Naturalized Bioethics: Toward Responsible Knowing and Practice (pp. 182–98). Cambridge: Cambridge University Press.

Tronto, J.C. (2013) *Caring Democracy, Markets, Equality and Justice*. New York: New York University Press.

Vaka, S., Brannelly, T. and Huntingdon, A. (2016) Getting to the heart of the story: using Talanoa to explore pacific mental health. *Issues in Mental Health Nursing*, 37(8), pp. 537–44. DOI: 10.1080/01612840.2016.1186253.

Walker, M.U. (2007) *Moral Understandings, A Feminist Study in Ethics*, 2nd edn. New York: Oxford University Press.

Young, I.M. (2006) Responsibility and global justice: a social connection model. *Social Philosophy and Policy*, 23, pp. 102–30, DOI: 10.1017/S0265052506060043.

3

Dilemmas of disclosure in mental health therapeutic education

Joanne Brown

Introduction

This chapter offers reflections on the place of one's personal voice in the context of mental health education (HE), based on over 25 years of experience of teaching and learning about mental health in higher education. I do not intend to prescribe a certain practice, but instead to discuss the place of one's personal voice in an academic context, which raises important ethical questions. This includes the questions of what is good for academics, for students and for service users when discussing experiences of mental distress in an academic context; what is an appropriate boundary in this place; and how we can be attuned to the reality of psychic distress without violating boundaries and being intrusive.

Although I do believe that we need a professional boundary or, in Winnicott's (1960) terms, an 'adaptive false self', I also think that we need to remind ourselves that this professional pretence is just that – even if we do not then continue to dismantle it. Personal experience can be acknowledged without disclosure, thus normalising psychic suffering and creating a conversational space in which we can interrogate what 'fitness to practise' and professionalism mean. It is important to do this in order that our personal voice is not shrouded in secrecy and shame, but acknowledged as existing and appropriately contained in our educational practices. Although I will point to the ethical issues which a silent personal voice raises, I am not arguing for academics and students to share more personal experience. There are many reasons why this might sometimes be ethically dubious, but what I do want to do is to point to the curious dynamic which is set up when we proceed as though academics and students do not have personal experiences of mental health difficulty. This potentially creates a situation in which academics and students feel as though they must deny their experience, and service users are asked to publicly disclose their personal experience of pain on our behalf. One of the questions this paper raises is whether this creates an 'us and them' mentality between academics and students on the one hand, and service users on the other. If this occurs, is it good for service users? Is it good for academics and students? And how do we address these asymmetries between groups? In mental health education, students are often asked to use who they are therapeutically in order to offer psychological contact and presence (in addition to other roles and responsibilities which they have) to the people they will work with. If, in our education, we have implicitly asked them to deny a part of who they are, how difficult might this task be?

This chapter presents reflections on three issues that are relevant, in my experience, to mental health education:

1. The silent, personal voice behind the public professional persona and the question of its appropriate role in informing teaching and learning about mental health.

2. Service user education and the possible perpetuation of an 'us and them' mentality in mental health education.

3. The difference between clinical and academic modes of teaching and learning, or states of mind, that the university setting uneasily combines.

These concerns, to my mind, are simultaneously ethical and pedagogical issues about educational practice. This chapter begins with a vignette about two academics talking about their recent struggles in their personal lives.

A vignette

Two 40-something women meet in a cafe. Rachel has been ill for weeks and is now suffering from post-viral fatigue. She has been referred for a scan, with a possible infection of the heart. The poignancy of having a possible infection of the heart is not lost on Sam, since she knows that Rachel has been in psychotherapy for a few years, trying to brave her inner demons and survive her brush with, what she sees as, the grim reaper of the emotional world – crushing, haunting and residing in those whose pain it feeds on. This psychic pain lives on the border between the mind and the body, and is visceral and bodily. 'I've been struggling lately,' Sam offers, knowing that this won't be met with pity, awkwardness or selfishness. 'What have you been feeling?' Rachel asks, not too soon, but not too late either – she doesn't rush in, but neither does she saunter too much. As Sam finds the words to say, she feels literally without hope; the pain wells up, fresh and pure. It's been underground for days, and there's a relief in letting it reach the surface. 'I can't say', she says. 'Why?' Rachel gently asks. 'I'll get upset', Sam says – the pain now ready to leave her body and give her some respite. The pressure eases and they talk about how to cope with their dual worlds of being private individuals and professional women – their personal and scholarly voices.

Silent, personal voices

Neither of them bring this personal voice to their work – not directly anyway – and it may be inappropriate to do so; but if their work involves learning and teaching about mental pain, does it set up a curious dynamic if their own pain has to be encased in professional competence and/or armour? If we dare not speak the name of pain as professionals, what kind of stigmatising of emotional suffering do we inadvertently perpetuate? I offer this as a point for discussion, not as a call to arms for all of those who are involved in teaching and learning about mental health to treat the classroom as a consulting room. I am psychodynamically trained, and boundaries are a central feature of psychodynamic work – perhaps sometimes too rigidly so, but I nevertheless see the importance of boundaries in terms of protecting ourselves, our clients, our students. As Coia (1999) points out, reflection on experience does not necessarily require a public demonstration, and she raises the ethical question of whether reflective forms of teaching and learning (e.g. diary-like personal journals) may be a violation of someone's privacy. Nevertheless, I think that we have a difficult situation for mental health staff and students who have to discuss, reflect on and try to help people with an excess of pain and damage in their lives, when they themselves might be harbouring and camouflaging their own.

And if they are, how do we know if it is because they are protecting their own privacy and/or out of a fear of being shamed? Hoggett (2017) explains that shame refers to a continuum of experience ranging from mild embarrassment to humiliation, and he argues that ours is a culture characterised by fear of shame. De Botton (2003, p. 112) argues that, in Christianity, we are seen as 'at heart, desperate, fragile creatures, a good deal less wise than we are knowledgeable, always on the verge of anxiety, tortured by our relationships, terrified of death'. This view of humanity as one beset by sources of suffering can be found in other world religions and philosophies. De Botton's aim is not to promote Christianity, but to argue that in education we should 'mine the works of great thinkers in order to help us understand better folly, envy, greed, pride, etc.' (De Botton, 2003) to which we are all subject. O'Neill (2014, p. 12) argues that we should 'write the hidden histories of academia' and 'think against the grain' and thus offer a way to 'disrupt the normative and usher in the space to think, feel, critique and change'. In health and social care education, this conjoining of the public and private voices is seen in auto-ethnography (Ellis, 2004; Short, Turner and Grant, 2013), and narrative is increasingly used as a form of recovery and social critique (see Frank, 1995; Deegan, 1988). Speaking about our personal struggles or doubts is not necessarily then, as Coia would caution against, promoting individualism, but an oppositional stance in relation to normative ideas about success.

The *Times Higher Education* magazine published a piece by Moran in 2015 that had an air of 'coming out' about it. Moran wrote about how it feels to be a shy academic in a sector which lives by the 'extrovert ideal' (see Cain's 'Quiet' [2013]). Moran did not bemoan the performative nature of the lecture, or the professional mask one might wear, but he did refer to the university as a 'motley family ... where very different personalities – shy, confident and all shades in between – can come together and feel at ease' (p. 35). Or, at least, this is what he was calling for. The so-called 'signature dilemma' (Geertz, 1988: the hidden, but powerful voice of the researcher in the social sciences) is one I have often wrestled with:

> I'm going to the last session of a module I teach on a two-year postgraduate course in mental health practice, and on my way up the stairs to twenty or so students. They have been a good, serious group of learners, hungry for psychological and less biomedical approaches to inpatient care. I feel apprehensive and my heartbeats as I hurriedly go to the room, armed with student evaluation forms. I notice the beating of my heart, and I identify it as fear, but I wonder what I'm afraid of. I catch it. I feel guilty. I feel like this deserving group of students could have been given more, but more of what? Of me, I think.

Three weeks into this course, I suffered a personal trauma, but I did not talk about it or want the students to feel like they had to look after my needs. But this raises the point about how we, as educators, might remain hidden or proceed as though we are people without biographies. I knew some of the students' difficulties (relationship breakdown, cancer, self-harm) and, of course, about their mental health practice where they were confronted with suicide, desperate need and violence. In one room, we therefore had the convergence of the facts of their lives and those of mine (some known and some hidden). A host of silent voices (see Fraiberg et al.

[1975], who wrote about uninvited guests from the past in every nursery) hovered around our discussions about mental health. My task, as a
mental health educator, was to think about how these life stories were
held (rather than split off and denied), without any of us becoming inap-
propriately confessional or conducting some 'wild analysis' (Freud, 1910)
in the classroom. Mental health students need to learn how to use who
they are therapeutically, and be grounded in themselves in order to do so.
On the above course, this was partly achieved by a 90-minute reflective
practice group unencumbered by learning outcomes, assessment methods
or outcome measures. It was one of the most valued aspects of the course
(see Brown, Simons and Zeeman, 2008).

However, what Finlay (2008) refers to as the 'dark side' of reflective
practice, along with the ethical questions it raises (about the risks of it
being coercively confessional, narcissistically indulgent and individual-
ised), is debated in the social sciences (Holt, 2003; Duncan, 2004; Ellis,
Adams and Bochner, 2011). In different schools of therapy, we also see
debates about whether and how much disclosure should be used in
practice, with related debates about the power differential that is insti-
tuted by boundaries and the notions of expertise which might surround
professionals (Frosh, 2015; Phillips, 1997). I have often felt a tension
between my psychodynamic training, with its emphasis on firm and containing boundaries around that which is personal, and the call for more
egalitarian relationships in mental health.

Those elected to speak

We have a tradition in health and social care, of course, of inviting
service users in to talk about their experience of being carers, clients and
patients. This development is informed by the idea of the 'expert by
experience' (DOH, 2001) and has led to recent attempts to co-produce
services, education and research (Loughran and Broderick, 2017;
Videmsek, 2017) with a view to assessing what impact on practice
these developments might have (Hughes, 2017; Grundy et al., 2017;
Terry, 2015). It is generally agreed that these innovations are important
attempts to humanise care (Feijoo-Cid et al., 2017).

Although these are invaluable developments, they do not necessarily address the way in which service users are asked to be the bearers of
psychic pain. Staff and students in healthcare education, for example,
might still be positioned as the people who do not have fractured lives
or suffer from, for example, depression or anxiety, and an 'us and them'
mentality might still prevail. Again, I must repeat that I am not calling for
a large-scale confessional among mental health professionals. Service user

involvement in higher education is an admirable attempt at inclusiveness, at de-stigmatising mental health problems. Indeed, I invite service users to teach on my courses every year, but does this carry a risk of giving service users the extraordinarily difficult job of carrying and speaking that which we as a society so fear?

There are important instances where celebrities, sportspeople, clinicians, politicians and so on come out and tell of their own personal struggles behind the professional role that they also inhabit. These can be important ways in which fallibility, weakness, vulnerability and shame can be seen to be struggles for those we might otherwise think of as only strong, successful and competent (Richards and Brown, 2001). Narratives from 'wounded healers' (Rippere and Williams, 1985) are democratising because they are very important reminders that clinicians and teachers are not exempt from the uncertainties, insecurities and losses that beset students, clients, friends and relatives. The transference to mental health teachers and/or clinicians can be very powerful because of the expertise we perhaps profess to have. If we are experts, for example on mental health problems, what is it that we profess to have a full working knowledge of, and is it theoretical and/or experiential? What is the source of my expertise on mental health – my battle with psychic suffering, my successful navigation out of it and/or my intellectual mastery of texts on mental health? And what fantasy do I help to perpetuate by silencing, if I do, my personal voice?

It is interesting, for example, to hear service users who have struggled with their own depression, messy relationships, history of abuse and so forth wonder if they might one day train to be mental health workers or counsellors, asking tentatively and with shame whether they would be allowed to do so. Similarly, students on mental health trainings (e.g. in mental health nursing) sometimes wonder whether they can admit to their own mental health difficulties when occupying the position of a nurse or counsellor. There is a reality, of course, to being well enough to train, but I think that when students ask this, it is a question inflected by the fantasies about and transferences towards mental health professionals that we can have.

Clinical and academic states of mind

Clearly, as mental health lecturers, we are not working as therapists for our students, and an educational context is not necessarily one in which to publicly process and work through our personal issues. However, it is a setting in which many of our personal issues may be consciously or unconsciously acted out, ameliorated, or denied. Moreover, mental health education demands that we learn more about who we are – for example how we learn, get close to or distance ourselves from people, behave in groups, feel about disclosure and so on (see Craib, 1994). And for this reason, some aspects of mental health teaching and learning require a different form of education that implicitly questions the acquisition of knowledge as a theoretical endeavour only.

In mental health nursing, Warne and McAndrew (2007) challenge 'the hegemonic value ... theoretical knowledge has acquired, particularly when the tenet of mental health practice is trying to understand and make sense of another's experiences of their psychic reality' (p. 227). They argue that the NHS performance-driven demand for evidence-based practice might paradoxically only serve to compromise the mental health nurses' ability to facilitate patient centredness (p. 226), because the thera-peutic relationship and co-presence are not easily objectively measured.

Hoggett (2017) argues that in post-industrial society, the impulse towards measurement and control has become ubiquitous, and he explains that 'some theorists now use the term epistemicide to describe the cognitive injustice involved in the marginalisation and, on occasion, extermination of different ways of knowing to those based upon measure-ment and calculability' (de Sousa Santos, 2014; Bennett, 2007).

Frosh (2015), from a psychoanalytic perspective, similarly bemoans the way in which in the neoliberal university knowledge has become compressed into 'a very particular model of utilitarianism' (p. 1). He argues that 'the belief that certain kinds of knowledge might produce psy-chological balance and be essential for a "good life" – that the search for such knowledge might indeed, be an ethical "good" in its own right and therefore be foundational for a good society – is quite outmoded' (p. 1). Although Frosh acknowledges that we need to demonstrate outcomes with the use of public money (student satisfaction, research impact, etc.), he also argues that the 'relentless insistence on productivity' limits and compresses what it might mean to know something. In a similar spirit, de Botton (2007) asks how knowledge can be used as a 'repertoire of wisdom' (p. 111) in the modern university.

Warne and McAndrew (2003) argue that nurse educators need 'to develop reflective and reflexive learning opportunities which are capa-ble of promoting profound uncertainty without losing the individual mental health nurse to anxiety, despair or resistance'. That is, 'nurses should question what underpins their practice and their competence to practise and work at the edges of knowing and not knowing' (p. 228). For them, this is possible through the recognition and value to be found in the nurse embracing the patient experience as a primary and legitimate source of knowledge (p. 228) rather than settling for 'a professional per-sona, which implicitly accepts the medical model'. Moreover, they argue that mental health nurses need to explore the intrapersonal relationships that exist between their self as a professional and person.

However, the competitive, rationalist, outcome-based form of health-care education in HE might not always be conducive to the kinds of learning that we need to facilitate in mental health: theoretical knowledge acquisition *and* personal and relational insight. If, for example, we want students to understand the aetiology and symptoms of borderline personality disorder, we need to introduce the personal voice of the service user via modes such as narrative, poetry and painting as well diagnostic criteria or attachment theories that might explain relational problems. And in addition to this, we need to help students to access their own personal experiences that either help or hinder them as they try to understand what it is like to have lived this person's life. This type of understanding, attunement or reflective skill is central to mental health education, and we all have different methods for fostering this clinical sensibility.

This type of understanding or clinical/reflective sensibility might mean that boisterous talkative students, who have an answer for most things, quieten down and struggle with not knowing for a while as they reach for understanding of themselves or the other. It might mean that the student who sees herself in the tragedy of the lives we present can find some appropriate distance, rather than run out of the room crying, or that the student who wants to have a laugh will be able to reside with tragedy a little more. That is, mental health teaching might require, as a necessary part of learning, a personal transformation or engagement with the habits of our personal voice (however privately) in order to really learn how to empathise or understand the lived experience of the people we work with.

In counselling or therapy trainings, students are often in therapy, looking at how their personal and professional lives are clashing, split, complementary and so on. However, students on most mental health trainings do not have recourse to this, if indeed they want it. However reflexive learning does exist in the form of reflective practice and clinical supervision (though it is something of a rare commodity in mental health practice). Reflective practice is a slow, meditative kind of work that often requires some humility as we look at some of the motives, actions and impulses at work or at play in our professional lives.

It might sometimes be hard for mental health teachers to find a genuine place for humility, modesty and critical reflectiveness in a very fast-paced, competitive HE setting, based on fantasies of invulnerability, knowledge and mastery. Honore's (2004) classic book *In Praise of Slow* challenged the 'cult of speed' in contemporary culture, and we now have a 'slow university' movement which is committed to finding a 'more reflective way of being, doing and living connected to addressing issues of well-being, the common good, connection and community' (O'Neill, 2014, p. 1).

Collective responsibility, care and support are, O'Neill explains, under-mined by competitive individualism and an audit culture. Hoggett refers to the self-tracking (audit of the self) culture as a phallic culture in which the self never measures up. Mountz et al. (2015) argue that a 'counting culture leads to intense, insidious forms of institutional shaming', and they refer to us making 'ourselves calculable rather than memorable' (p. 1243). Moreover, they ask, 'What if we counted differently? Instead of articles published or grants applied for, what if we accounted for thank you notes received, friendships formed, collaborations forged?' (p. 1243). This reframing of the curriculum vitae (CV) recalls Gusdorf's (1980) ironic claim that the CV can become an apology for living and 'theodicy of being'. Whether one agrees with Mountz et al.'s alternative 'performance' meas-ures (they could usher in their own competitive ethic) is beside the point. They are cited because they are trying to think about how the philosophy and values base which underpins education can be critically questioned.

In their work on the slow university, Mountz et al. argue for the need for a feminist ethics of care in the sector, pointing out that 'care work is work. It is not self-indulgent' (p. 1238). Marginalising care, they argue, 'furthers the myth that we are autonomous individuals (Lawson, 2007) and they state that care is a political activity when practised in institu-tions which devalue it' (p. 1239).

Although reflective practice may be central to being a balanced or integrated mental health teacher and to understanding a client's life, it might not pay observable dividends. For example, it might not lead to prolific publications, conference papers, successful bids, protocols or measurable outcomes, and it is therefore a kind of devalued emotional labour in higher education. However, in clinical psychotherapeutic practice, we might be 'taught' to be vigilant about our more omnipotent, narcissistic and competitive blind spots in order to protect clients from the clinician acting out his or her own needs, problems and wishes.

Of course some critical theorists (Furedi, 2003; Ecclestone and Hayes, 2009) bemoan the 'rise of dangerous therapeutic education' because it positions the learner as vulnerable and leads to a lowering of academic standards. There isn't space here to converse with their argument in detail, but it is important to point out that a reflective mental health education can be combined with an academically rigorous training. Moreover, it does not position the learner as debilitated, but as resil-ient and strong enough to contact his or her own vulnerability without collapsing. Without this personal work, empathy would be extraordinar-ily difficult in practice.

Emotional reflexive labour is therefore central to learning in most psychotherapeutic trainings. The fruits of this labour might be seen in a client feeling a little more understood, less alone, isolated or ashamed. Sam, in the above example, felt relieved of the pressure of a pain borne alone when Rachel, someone with understanding, knew how to ask what was wrong and knew how to listen and grasp something of Sam's experience. This simple exchange (Rachel knowing how to inquire, understand psychic terror, use the self therapeutically, etc.) requires a particular clinical state of mind that might not be easy to hold onto in our busy institutional lives in which there is a competition for recognition, power, status and resources. In the context of HE, this clinical or reflective state of mind is sometimes antithetical to the competitive noise to which we are all subject as we look ahead to the Research Excellence Framework (REF), publications, bids, or Nursing and Midwifery Council (NMC) visits which do not necessarily draw on capacities for modesty, productive inaction and a reflection on our personal struggles.

Conclusion

At the end of the two-year postgraduate course mentioned above, one student had the idea to bring in coloured card and envelopes. We were all to take small pieces of card and write something about each member of the group and put it in the envelope with the person's name on it. The cards that I read, and still have 10 years later, are testimony to what a personal journey mental health education can be. The messages are generous, tongue-in-cheek and moving ('keep the fire burning', 'I feel like a new person', 'where do you buy your skirts?'). But one of the messages which is relevant to this discussion read 'Thank you for bringing something of yourself'.

Although there are challenges to teaching and learning about mental health in HE, it is possible to keep our personal and scholarly voices on parallel tracks without necessarily disclosing private pain or electing other people to exclusively embody it. For example, I try to stay close to my memories and experiences of fear, exclusion, irrationality, shame and loneliness when I teach and learn about psychic suffering, without necessarily disclosing details. In this way, I stay near to the subject at hand and look inwards and outwards simultaneously. I look inwards to my own private struggles and out to other lives and the world of scholarship that tries to understand and analyse them. In this way, I hope that my personal and scholarly voices do not become akin to divergent tracks between which I must choose, but neither do they chaotically collapse into each other. Rather, they remain parallel and attuned.

This chapter has not set out to prescribe how or whether personal and scholarly voices should be conjoined in mental healthcare education. It has pointed to the problematic nature of keeping a personal voice completely hidden, leaving service users with the task of bearing and speaking the name of psychic pain when some of us (students and lecturers) also know how this feels. The dilemmas of disclosure and the 'dark side' of reflective practice have been discussed, and the context in which we try to learn about psychic life and relationships has been highlighted in order to ask whether it is a context which can contain reflective practice and value different forms of knowledge. Although, as advocates of the slow university movement claim, it might be politically important to bring something of our authentic selves to the workplace (Mountz et al., 2015), the question of how this is done in mental health education is both a pedagogical and ethical issue which each of us might need unhurried time to think about.

References

Bennett, K. (2007) Epistimicide! *The Translator*, 31(2), pp. 152–69.

Brown, J., Simons, L. and Zeeman, L. (2008) New ways of working in Mental Health: Practitioner views of their training and role. *Journal of Psychiatric and Mental Health Nursing*, 15(10), pp. 823–32.

Cain, L. (2013) *Quiet: The Power of Introverts in a World that Can't Stop Talking*. London: Broadway Books.

Coia, L. (1999) Reflections on writing autobiographically in the classroom. *Inquiry: Critical Thinking Across the Disciplines*, 18(3), pp. 12–25.

Craib, I. (1994) *The Importance of Disappointment*. London: Routledge.

de Botton, A. (2003) *Religion for Atheists: A Non-Believer's Guide to the Uses of Religion*. London: Vintage.

Deegan, P.E. (1988) Recovery: The lived experience of rehabilitation. *Psychosocial Rehabilitation Journal*, 11(4), pp. 11–19.

de Sousa Santos, B., (2014) *Another Knowledge is Possible: Beyond Northern Epistemologies*. London: Verso.

DOH (2001) *The Expert Patient: A New Approach to Chronic Disease Management for the 21st Century*. London: HMSO.

Duncan, M. (2004), Autoethnography: Critical appreciation of an emerging art. *International Journal of Qualitative Methods*, 3(4), pp. 28–39.

Ecclestone, K. and Hayes, D. (2009) *The Dangerous Rise of Therapeutic Education*. London: Routledge.

Ellis, C. (2004) *The Ethnographic I: A Methodological Novel about Autoethnography*. Lanham, MD: AltaMira Press.

Ellis, C. Adams, T.E., Bochner, A.P. (2011) Autoethnography: An overview. *Historical Social Research*, 36(4), pp. 273–90.

Feijoo-Cid, M. Morina, D., Gomez-Ibanez, R. and Leyva-Moral, J.M. (2017) Expert patient illness narratives as a teaching methodology: A mixed method study of student nurses satisfaction. *Nurse Education Today*, 50, pp. 1–7.

Finlay, L. (2008) Reflecting on reflective practice, Practice-based Professional Learning (PBPL) Centre paper, 52.

Fraiberg, S., Adelson, E. and Shapiro, V. (1975) Ghosts in the nursery: A psycho-analytic approach to the problems of impaired mother–infant relationships. *Journal of the American Academy of Child Psychiatry*, 14(3), pp. 387–421.

Frank, A. (1995) *The Wounded Storyteller: Body, Illness and Ethics*. London and Chicago, IL: The University of Chicago Press.

Freud, S. (1957) *The Standard Edition of the Complete Psychological Works of Sigmund Freud: Five lectures on psycho-analysis, Leonardo Da Vinci and other works*, Volume 11 (1910) London: Hogarth Press.

Frosh, S. (2015) You leave here stamped, 'credit points', Psychoanalysis and Education Conference (22–24 October), The School of Education, University of Sheffield in association with The Northern School of Child and Adolescent Psychotherapy.

Furedi, F. (2003) *Therapy Culture: Cultivating Vulnerability in an Age of Uncertainty*. London: Routledge.

Geertz, C. (1988) *Works and Lives: The Anthropologist as Author*. Stanford, CA: Stanford University Press.

Grundy, A.C., Walker, L., Meade, O., Fraser, C., Cree, L., Bee, P., Lovell, K. and Callaghan, P. (2017) Evaluation of a co-delivered training package for community mental health professionals on service user- and carer-involved care planning. *Journal of Psychiatric and Mental Health Nursing*, 24(6) pp. 358–66.

Gusdorf, G. (1980) Conditions and limits of autobiography, in Olney, J. (Ed.), *Autobiography: Essays Theoretical and Critical* (pp. 28–48). Princeton, NJ: Princeton University Press.

Hoggett, P. (2017) Shame and performativity: Thoughts on the psychology of neoliberalism. *Psychoanalysis, Culture and Society*, 22(4) 364–82.

Holt, N.L. (2003) Representation, legitimation and autoethnography: An autoethnographic writing story. *International Journal of Qualitative Methods*, 2(1), pp. 18–28.

Honore, C. (2004) *In Praise of Slow: How a Worldwide Movement is Challenging the Cult of Speed*. London: Orion Books.

Hughes, M. (2017) What difference does it make? Findings of an impact study of service user and carer involvement on social work students' subsequent practice. *Social Work Education*, 36(2), pp. 203–16 .

Lawson, R. (2007) Home and hospital: Hospice and palliative care: How the environment impacts the social work role. *Journal of Social Work in End of Life and Palliative Care*, 3(2), pp. 3–17.

Loughran, H. and Broderick, G. (2017) From service-user to social work examiner: Not a bridge too far. *Social Work Education*, 36(2), pp. 188–202 .

Moran, J. (2015) The Quiet Life, in *Times Higher Education*, September, 2015, pp. 31–35.

Mountz, A., Bonds, A., Mansfield, B., Loyd, J., Hyndman, J. and Walton-Roberts, M. (2015) For slow scholarship: A feminist politics of resistance through collective action in the neoliberal university. *ACME – An International E-Journal for Critical Geographies*, 14(4), pp. 1235–59.

O'Neill, M. (2014) The slow university: Work, time and well-being. *Forum: Qualitative Social Research*, 15(3), pp. 1–20.

Phillips, A. (1997) *Terrors and Experts*. Cambridge, MA: Harvard University Press.

Richards, B. and Brown, J. (2001) Media as drivers of the therapeutic trend? *Free Associations*, 62, pp. 18–30.

Rippere, V. and Williams, R. (eds). (1985) *Wounded Healers*. London: John Wiley and Sons.

Short, N.P., Turner, L. and Grant, A. (eds). (2013) *Contemporary British Autoethnography*. Rotterdam/Boston/Tapei: Sense Publishers.

Terry, J. (2015) Service user involvement in pre-registration mental health nurse education classroom settings: A review of the literature. *Journal of Psychiatric and Mental Health Nursing*, 19, 816–29.

Videmsek, P. (2017) Expert by experience research as grounding for social work education. *Social Work Education*, 36(2), pp. 172–87.

Warne, T. and McAndrew, S. (2007) Passive patient or engaged expert? Using a Ptolemaic approach to enhance mental health nurse education and practice. *International Journal of Mental Health Nursing*, 16, pp. 224–229.

Winnicott, D.W. (1960). Ego distortion in terms of true and false self, in Winnicott, D.W. (ed.). (1965), *The Maturational Process and the Facilitating Environment: Studies in the Theory of Emotional Development* (pp. 140–52). London: Hogarth Press and the Institute of Psychoanalysis.

4

Time to reflect: relationships and ethics

David Woods and Roger Ingham

Discussion

A public sector that demands reliable, measurable, high-quality outcomes from well-integrated, well-functioning professional and interprofessional teams of healthcare practitioners and educators in a fast-paced, productive work environment – is this hyper-benign description simply a reflection of our modernised healthcare system, the reality of which we have little choice but to accept? Or is it instead an overly simplistic, top-down ideal whose misconceived and incoherent aims end up exerting a serious moral strain upon those who are ultimately responsible for delivering it? The picture that emerges from the chapters in this section would seem to point to the latter. According to Engward and Papanikitas, for instance, it cannot be taken as a given that interprofessional teams can get to work in the manner required above without at least some consideration of how to negotiate and co-ordinate between the various different professional codes, values and principles represented in any given team. Indeed, according to Brown, the thick veneer of professionalism itself may obstruct the kinds of outcomes that a truly ideal healthcare system ought to provide. Such an ideal healthcare system, Brannelly proposes, would be unlike the one described above insofar as it would not be defined and measured in purely operational terms – where the service user, positioned as external to the system, is inputted at one end and emerges as an outcome at the other – but instead in terms of the intrinsically relational, and intrinsically ethical, notion of care.

By raising these issues, the chapters in this section offer some initial guidance for how to conceptualise, manage and perhaps even challenge the everyday demands put on healthcare professionals by the healthcare system itself. Because the title of this section indicates *emerging* debates in healthcare ethics, however, many more questions and difficulties are raised than can possibly be answered all in one go. In this brief discussion, we aim to bring some of these questions and difficulties to the surface and to outline one way of beginning to explore them in an educational setting.

To start, Brown argues that, for too long, healthcare professionals, whether they be practitioners or educators (or both), have felt the need to silence their personal voices for the sake of their professional personas. Instead, she suggests that professionals should, where appropriate, feel able to draw upon and share relevant personal experience. What are the possible ethical reasons for sharing personal experience in the education and/or work environment? One reason Brown suggests is that it would be duplicitous not to; failure to acknowledge that professionals – who are, after all, people too – are equally capable of falling victim to the same maladies about which they dispassionately theorise, perpetuates a divisive 'us and them' mentality. A second reason, this time from the perspective of our relationships *within* the professional sphere, is that we ought to fight against a 'put up and shut up' culture where professionals – again, people too – feel unable to break through the shell of their own out- wardly 'coping' personae. Finally, of course, in the right circumstances, the ability and freedom to share or draw upon personal experience might enable us, as professionals, to produce new and better outcomes in healthcare and education.

But what about the possible ethical reasons for professionals *not* to share their personal experiences? Here we find ourselves in the grip of moral uncertainties which are probably responsible for our initial instinct to keep silent. As Brown notes, when educators begin sharing personal experiences (or even deep feelings), there is the risk that the education process acquires an overly confessional tone; it could end up putting pressure on educators and, of course, students to reveal some deeply personal things about themselves. Moreover, the professional persona is arguably not just there for the protection of the professional; it is also there to protect those for whom the professional has assumed respon- sibility. After all, it can be burdensome to know personal information about someone else. What are students to do should they learn – or recognise – for instance, that their tutor suffers from anxiety or shows stress-related behaviours? Is it incumbent on them to alter their own expectations or adapt their approach – or might we expect them to cope with the recognition that vulnerability is simply part of being human? And need we assume that being human, and at times subject to ailments and afflictions, means we are any less able to do the work, whether of education or healthcare?

Of course professionals need a professional environment in which to be people too. But, given the possible ethical risks of liberating the personal voice in the ways outlined above, and in spite of the appreciable possible benefits, a final, wider question presents itself: are we in danger of promoting a rhetoric of trust and respect for whole people who have needs and strengths and care about others, while in our actions colluding with an agenda that promotes only individual survival and achievement?

Like Brown, the other contributors to this section also raise ethical questions about relationships, their boundaries and the manifold difficulties associated with observing, transgressing, adjusting and, in some cases, dismantling these boundaries. In the case of Engward and Papanikitas, who focus on the relationships between different professional groupings, the ethical boundaries are determined by (sometimes) substantial differences in professional principles, structures and processes. Until such differences are acknowledged and sufficiently understood, they can remain as obstacles to enhanced patient care. But given that these differences are as limitless as the different possible interprofessional combinations in any given team, each team must achieve the requisite mutual understanding for itself (if it does at all). Once again, therefore, the unavoidable everyday ethical challenges of healthcare work do not appear to be immediately compatible with any ideal that simply takes for granted speed, integration and functionality. And yet, presumably, such ideals are not devised in a vacuum and imposed for their own sake; they are themselves the responses of a healthcare system under very real external pressures – social, political, economic and otherwise.

Brannelly, who focuses on the relationship between practitioners and service users, has an expressly radical proposal. Rather than using understanding to *reach across* established boundaries, Brannelly proposes that a certain type of understanding aimed at the service user and associated with care ethics (the ethical theory that, according to Brannelly, gives us the most appropriate ethical guidance for healthcare policy and provision), demands a radical *revision* – perhaps even *demolition* – of the established boundaries between practitioners and service users. In her empirical research, Brannelly finds that use of compulsion in the treatment of mental illness, in particular, highlights the problematic nature of these boundaries. The message that Brannelly receives loud and clear is that mental health service users strongly favour the abolition of compulsion, primarily because it establishes a power inequality with far-reaching detrimental consequences for the quality and outcomes of mental healthcare provision, including dis-incentivising people in serious need from seeking help, for fear of being compelled, and ultimately raising doubts and suspicions about whose interests are prioritised in the decision to compel – those of the service user or those of the general public (supposedly) at risk. This on top of the fact that the unique and often lucid insight of service users into their own conditions and situations,

Brannelly finds, is overlooked by healthcare policies that appear to be designed to work *against* service users rather than *with* them.

Of course, presumably, one could aim to construct a care ethics argument *in favour* of compulsion on the grounds that the necessity of compulsion may in certain cases follow even from a genuinely caring attitude towards the service user. Indeed, possibly, such an argument could be constructed on the grounds that a genuinely caring attitude towards the general public may, unfortunately, require the compelled treatment of an individual member of the public, such as seclusion and restraint, in which case protectionism, on the one hand, and care, on the other, would not appear to be forever at odds; sometimes, one derives from the other. But this seems wide of Brannelly's point. The point may not be that care ethics *necessarily* rules out all forms of compulsion, seclusion, restraint and protectionism. Rather, the point may be that if the viewpoint of the service user were taken more seriously than it is now (which, Brannelly argues, according to care ethics it should be), then the challenge to these methods and the policies designed around them (which, Brannelly finds, issues from that viewpoint) must also be taken seriously.

Perhaps the best way to achieve an understanding of all of these different contributors – the educator, the student, the professional, the practitioner, the service user and, of course, the person concealed behind them all – is to try inhabiting them. Redolent of Brown's chapter, we may inhabit several already and find it relatively straightforward to think flexibly about different perspectives. Active approaches to discussing and rehearsing different possible scenarios involving perspective-taking can raise concrete, specific difficulties that emerge from the relationships and boundaries between them, on the one hand, and at the same time help to develop the kind of mutual understanding which could contribute to solving these difficulties, on the other. Discussion can focus on justifications for viewpoints, assertions and decisions in order to enable the basic ethical substrates – the 'taken-for-granted' assumptions – of perspectives to be identified and explored. It is not crucial to arrive at a clear solution to the dilemmas; indeed, the success of such experiential learning is claimed if we are better able to consider the dynamic processes through which our own – and others' – decisions are reached, which will hopefully stand us all in good stead when faced with new ethical care and purely pragmatic challenges as working lives unfold. Achieving this may be the biggest challenge of all – the current obsession with efficiency, measurement and outputs risks diminishing the space for reflection on the real purpose of healthcare, and the central role that human relationships play in achieving excellence.

PART 2

Changing Practices

Better Than This[1,2]

Molly Case

I

Baby and me are only three months together,
brought through storm clouds
and rainbows and April-shower weather.
The decision I made,
whether to have her or not,
was based entirely on this marvellous brain that I've got,
full of colours and shadows and cracks in the surface,
that only some can reach.
And I listened to politicians on the news speak
of decisions on mental health provisions
that were hard to make,
fake feelings to disguise underhand dealings
like cutting beds.
All I want to know is there will be somebody
there to look after me,
if I need,
a hand to hold,
a safe bed to lie in and rest my head

---

[1] We have all seen the negative effects on our health and social care system in recent years, marred by harsh cuts and understaffing. I wrote this poem to give a voice to the people who often go unheard, the people we meet and help to treat every day, so affected by their circumstances, their living conditions, their mental health, their lack of income. When the Grenfell tragedy happened, I knew I wanted this poem to be heard widely. We all deserve to be listened to: our society must do better than this. MC.

[2]

when all my thoughts are hanging loose,
like unravelling threads.
'Cos I can't bear the thought
of stormy minds like mine
left to wander alone in the rain instead.

II

The rain doesn't bother me:
I like the smell it leaves on the bark of the tree.
For one whole year I have had HIV –
one year of becoming less and less like me
and not because of the disease,
but the way people are treating me.
When work found out they sent me a letter
asking me to take annual leave,
I've overheard colleagues already grieving for me,
perceiving me to be too sick to do my work.
What if the doctor thinks like that too?
What if there's a cost for medication?
God knows what I'll do.
What if the clinic treats me the same?
I guess I'll just stay out here,
with the trees and the rain.

III

Monday morning;
curtain open just enough
to see the rainclouds through.
On the table;
food vouchers and emergency food,
who'd have thought I'd be reliant on these phrases.
Days pass and my fridge holds nothing,
electricity and gas
buzzing and warm this week,
but my stomach is a hard, hollow shell
weak at the smell of warm soup and baked bread.
This hunger is so forceful I go for days just lying in bed.

IV

In my front room, waiting again.
Rain braids the living room window,
don't know
if carers are coming today,
if not I'll have to stay in this room
watching the world turn grey.
Some say I should just move to a care home
but I want to live here,
with all my old photographs,
and my books that have been here for years.
I thought our hopes & fears
were protected by clear guidelines:
the right to healthcare, to food,
a safe home to live,
a place to grow old and
sit and reminisce.
There are rights to being human
and to a life that's better than this.

5

Moving beyond the 'yuk' factor: ethical issues in breastmilk sharing and donation

Sally Dowling

Introduction

This chapter examines the way in which practices relating to informal breastmilk sharing and donation raise ethical issues for healthcare practitioners and breastfeeding supporters. Human milk is given for use by others in both regulated and unregulated ways; here these practices are contrasted and questions asked about the nature of donation – for example whether donors and recipients are viewed differently according to the mode of donation (milk bank vs milk sharing; donating vs selling) and the situation of the recipient. A range of approaches to thinking about these issues is outlined – drawing on ideas about other forms of bodily donation, cultural perceptions of women's bodies and their fluids, and ethical and legal approaches to body ownership. Issues raised include these questions: is the ethics of 'giving' a body product different when the product is human milk rather than blood or organs? Is this an area which should remain unregulated, as a private practice, or should it be more widely or formally considered? Can, or should, we regulate women's support for one another using their bodies?

The primary focus here is on informal milk sharing as an 'everyday health and care practice' – why and how it happens and how both donation and risk are framed and accounted for. Issues for both professionals (midwives, health visitors and nurses) and non-professionals (paid and unpaid breastfeeding supporters) working with pregnant and lactating women will also be raised. Milk sharing outside of formal milk banking arrangements is an emerging field of academic enquiry; some of this recent work will be used to illustrate this discussion. UK-related issues are the focus, but very little research has been undertaken in this area in the

UK, and so the chapter also draws on information and research from other countries. The intention is not to provide answers (and many questions are raised), but to increase awareness of the issues and to stimulate debate.

Background

Why give babies donated breastmilk?

Breastmilk is the optimal source of nutrition for babies, providing health benefits for mothers (Victora et al., 2016), and economic and other advantages for society (Pokhrel et al., 2015; Rollins et al., 2016). The World Health Organisation (WHO) recommends that all babies are fed on their mother's milk exclusively (i.e. no other food or fluids) for six months and then that breastfeeding continues, alongside other foods, for at least two years (WHO/UNICEF, 2003). These recommendations are based on good, regularly updated evidence and are for both developing and developed countries (e.g. see Victora et al., 2016). If a mother is unable to feed her baby from her breast, the WHO suggests that 'best alternatives' include breastmilk from a healthy wet nurse and breastmilk from a milk bank (WHO/UNICEF, 2003). Feeding with artificial breastmilk substitutes ('formula' milk) is the least advisable; this is because of the known negative outcomes for health (Victora et al., 2016). There are a range of situations in which breastfeeding might be difficult for those who want to breastfeed; these include prematurity but may also be due to the baby or the mother being unwell, or the mother having had breast or other surgery. There are also many socially influenced reasons: for example pressures to return to work, perceived milk insufficiency and/ or a lack of personal and cultural support. Social and cultural support are recognised as crucial in enabling women to establish and maintain breastfeeding and are particularly pertinent issues in the UK; these have been the focus of recent publications (Rollins et al., 2016; McFadden et al., 2017) and campaigns (UNICEF UK, 2016).

Across time, and around the world, women have engaged in informal breastmilk-sharing arrangements, often with friends or family – what Shaw calls 'cross-nursing' (Shaw, 2004, 2007). Formal wet-nursing arrangements have also existed, often determined by class and race issues; wealthy women around the world have paid others to breastfeed their babies (Palmer, 2009) and the history of breastfeeding for African American women is complicated by accounts of slave women breastfeeding their masters' babies (West and Knight, 2017). Why might a woman in the UK want to donate milk or to feed another woman's baby? Many women find that, once breastfeeding their own infant is established, they have an excess supply of milk (Geraghty et al., 2011). Alongside this, cheaper, easily available breast pumps; refrigeration; and a cultural expectation of pumping (Hausman, 2004; Geraghty et al., 2005; Stearns, 2010; Boyer, 2014) mean that many women have more breastmilk than their own baby needs.[1] There may be a reluctance to throw this away and a desire to help other women who may not have enough milk or who have babies who are premature or unwell (Cassidy, 2012). Occasionally, the death of a baby at or around birth may also lead a woman to want to donate the milk she makes (Welborn, 2012).

Why might babies need donor breastmilk? There are both physiological and social reasons. Babies who are premature or unwell need to be fed with breastmilk; the risk of necrotising enterocolitis (NEC) and other infections is high (and very serious) for premature babies, but breastmilk is also important for those with infections or other difficulties, as breastmilk is easier to digest. The mother may have died or be seriously unwell, have had a mastectomy or other surgery or is being treated with medication incompatible with breastfeeding. She may have returned to work and be unable to express milk there or be unable to express enough to maintain her supply. She may wish for her child to receive breastmilk exclusively until six months – as per WHO guidance – but circumstances, including those outlined above, may make this difficult.

Milk banking

The development of organised milk banking provision arose in many countries during the twentieth century (see Swanson, 2014),[2] but many closed during the 1980s due to concerns about blood-borne viruses, including HIV. A number re-emerged again over time, following advances in testing and treatment of donated milk. These were often, in the UK, in relation to local campaigns and charitable fundraising, although NHS England is now funding one regional bank, in South West England, in a model which may spread throughout the UK. One milk bank in the UK, in Queen Charlotte's and Chelsea Hospital, London, has been continuously operating since 1939. Some are also involved in scientific research using breastmilk, including in relation to environmental concerns and breast cancer.

---

[1] This is mainly written about in relation to the United States; the issues for women in the UK are likely to be very similar.

[2] This is a good description of how this came about in the United States: there is currently no equivalent history for the UK.

Milk banking exists in different forms around the world; in some, donors are paid, and recipient families pay for milk; in many, milk is donated for free, and in some, milk is available free of cost. In countries like the United States, without universal healthcare, there is often a cost for breastmilk. In the UK, the network of human milk banks receives donations from unpaid donors and distributes milk, free of cost to the parents, via the National Health Service (NHS), primarily to premature and sick infants, supported by National Institute for Health and Care Excellence (NICE) guidance (NICE, 2010) and the UK Association for Milk Banking (UKAMB). These milk banks are operated in different ways, and variations in geographical spread and funding mean that women who want to donate or receive breastmilk are not always able to do so. Milk banks only take breastmilk from women whose babies are healthy, have not yet been weaned and who are under six months of age. They are not able to take milk from women who smoke or use illegal drugs or some prescription medications, have tested positive for a range of blood-borne viruses (including Hepatitis B and C, HIV and syphilis) or who have had a blood transfusion (NICE, 2010; UKAMB, 2016a). Discourse around the ethics of the provision and use of human milk in this way often emphasises issues of risk and safety and of institutional responsibility; UKAMB and the NICE Guideline focus on these issues in relation to how donated milk is tested, transported and stored (including labelling and tracking so that it is always possible to know whom the milk has come from and which baby it has been given to), who should and who should not donate milk, how donors should be screened and who should receive donated milk (NICE, 2010; UKAMB, 2016a).

Milk sharing

In the UK, as in many other countries, full-term healthy babies are rarely eligible for banked milk. However, as noted above, there may be women who want to give their babies more breastmilk or for a longer period of time than they are able to themselves. Consequently, ways of donating informally have developed, often using the terminology of 'sharing', usually to full-term infants. Some women feed one another's babies via friendship groups while others contact one another using online (often international) networks specifically set up for the purpose of peer-to-peer human milk sharing, using websites, Facebook and Twitter to facilitate contacts. Akre et al. (2011) note that the use of the internet and social media has facilitated the transition of milk sharing from *'private practice to public pursuit'*. The two main networks, to date, have been 'Eats on Feets' and 'Human Milk 4 Human Babies', although there are also local examples.

Discussion – what are the issues?

What are the health risks in sharing breastmilk?

Several different terms have been used in the literature to describe sharing breastmilk online, including 'peer-to-peer milk sharing' (Gribble, 2013), 'peer milk sharing' (Carter and Reyes-Foster, 2016) and 'milky matches' (Cassidy, 2012); 'private arrangement milk sharing' and 'community breastmilk sharing' are also used on milk sharing websites. Most of these are international, athough some have local 'chapters'; there are also specifically local groups, often set up via Facebook for example. These terms emphasise the supportive, cooperative nature of the exchange. Sharing breastmilk via the internet is different to milk sharing among friends, although there are many similarities; the way the practice has arisen and developed can be seen to be a form of 'mother-to-mother' support, in much the same way as many breastfeeding support organisations have arisen (e.g. La Leche League, internationally, and the Association of Breastfeeding Mothers and the Breastfeeding Network in the UK). Seeing it as an 'act of care', in the same way as breastfeeding one's child might be seen, is another way of conceptualising the practice (Carroll, 2015); in this way it can also be thought of as an 'everyday' act. In the UK, we have no way of knowing how much milk sharing is happening, although recent research in the United States has attempted to find out more about both how common this is as well as about how women assess, and mitigate against, potential risks (Palmquist and Doehler, 2014, 2015). This was found to include gaining information about the donor woman such as whether is she still breastfeeding, how she expresses and stores the milk, whether she has been tested for a range of conditions, and so on. Donor mothers and recipient mothers often meet one another; receiving milk from completely unknown donors is unusual.

Although breastmilk is also **sold** via the internet – (not just to those seeking milk for babies but also for adult consumption), with one site asking recently, 'Are you over producing and want to list your liquid gold for sale?' (Only the Breast, 2017) – this is beyond the scope of this chapter. The focus here is on breastmilk sharing, defined as

> the commerce free practice in which a donor gives milk directly to a recipient family for the purpose of infant feeding or breastfeeds a recipient infant.
>
> (Palmquist and Doehler, 2015, p. 1)

Public health bodies in a number of countries have issued warnings against obtaining breastmilk in this way (either for money or for free), focusing usually on 'danger' and 'risk' (the US Food and Drug

Administration [FDA], Health Canada and the Agency for the Hygiene Safety of Health Products in France (AFSSAPS) are three examples). In the UK, there has been no advice on this from the Department of Health or Public Health England; some breastfeeding support organisations and the UKAMB have statements on their websites about milk sharing, but these usually focus on reducing risk and on emphasising the benefits of milk banks (e.g. LLL GB, 2017; UKAMB, 2016b).

The topics of milk sharing and selling as growing practices, and the potential risks associated with this, have been the subject of a range of academic papers as well as discussions online and in the media, raising questions about the ethical issues and obligations in this area. The concern of health bodies is usually expressed as being about the risk of contamination and infection, although to a certain extent these risks are unknown. The relative safety of milk sharing is usually compared to formula milk or to banked donor milk. Gribble and Hausman (2012), comparing the risks to using formula milk, point out that using artificial milk substitutes carries an increased risk of non-infectious diseases, gastro-intestinal disease and respiratory infections and contamination – and yet this is very common and rarely questioned. A limited amount of research has attempted to quantify the risks of obtaining breastmilk online (Cohen et al., 2009; Keim et al., 2013, 2014, e.g.) although this has focused on analysing milk for sale via the internet rather than milk donated via milk-sharing online organisations. Drawing on this small body of research (and often not distinguishing between whether milk is for sale or donated free, or if the donor is known or unknown) negatively loaded terms have been used about the practice:

> ... sharing a body fluid ... is dangerous ... playing Russian Roulette with your child's life ...
>
> (Updegrove, 2013, quoted in Palmquist, 2015);

> ... these women who are doing this are going to hurt, even kill, their babies ...
>
> (McCann, 2013, quoted in Palmquist, 2015); and

> ... breastmilk holds many known benefits, seeking out another's milk rather than turning to instant formula poses risks ...
>
> (Steele et al., 2015a)

There are undoubtedly some *potential* risks inherent in sharing breastmilk, both viral and bacterial, including the risks of contamination from handling. Research from the United States suggests that women seeking breastmilk online make careful judgements about risks (Palmquist and Doehler, 2015), asking lifestyle and health screening questions as part of the process of getting to know the milk donor. Evidence suggests that breastmilk is mostly sought for full-term infants and that the use of milk obtained via the internet (from strangers) often happens alongside milk sharing/cross-nursing with known women. Milk-sharing websites and the women using them often talk about how they exercise 'informed choice' – before breastmilk is obtained all the available evidence about potential risk is examined, and information is shared about safe collection, home pasteurisation and storage (Eats on Feets, 2017). If there is a concern about a specific risk, the donor woman may be asked screening questions about that risk. Often a woman obtaining milk in this way does not feel that the donor is a stranger, as quite a lot of information may be exchanged first, as noted above, including whether the donor woman is still breastfeeding her own baby. And there will often be continued contact between donors and recipients. These may include, for example, emails, phone calls, the exchange of photographs or meeting in person (Palmquist and Doehler, 2015).

One way of dealing with the unknown, but possible, risks inherent in sharing breastmilk outside a regulated system would be to invest in the milk banking network in the UK, increase the number of donors and relax the regulations, to make breastmilk universally available to every baby or child who was felt to need it – for medical, social or other reasons. It is unlikely that this will happen; many milk banks experience periodic shortages of donors (and therefore of supply) and premature and unwell babies would always be prioritised. In the UK, social pressure to wean soon after six months, despite the WHO guidance, means that breastfeeding into the second year of life or beyond is unusual (Dowling and Brown, 2013); anyone seeking breastmilk for a baby in this age range is unlikely to receive social approval. Research in the United States suggests that, at present, women who donate to breastmilk banks are a different group to those who share their milk informally and via other arrangements (Palmquist and Doehler, 2015). But, as we know that breastmilk is the optimal way to feed babies and young children, it could be argued that it is unethical not to facilitate ways to make breastmilk available to the many and not just the few. This could be seen as a public health responsiblity, although there would be competition for scarce resources, along with other issues that could be perceived as public health priorities.

How are regulated and unregulated milk donation perceived?

Breastmilk is culturally constructed in often confusing and contrasting ways – seen as both pure and dirty (Dowling et al., 2012). There are associations with pollution, danger and 'matter out of place' (Hausman,

2011; Douglas, 1966); these also relate to the ways in which women's bodies and other bodily fluids are seen. Societal expectations reinforce discretion and the hiding of breastmilk leakage (Dowling and Pontin, 2017; Zizzo, 2011). Milk donated to milk banks, subsequently used to help sick or premature babies, is often talked and written about in different terms to those used to describe milk shared via the internet – 'pure gold' vs 'fools gold', for example (Carter and Reyes-Foster, 2016). As noted above, the way in which milk sharing is written about is often alarmist, contrasting 'safe' (regulated) with 'dangerous' (unregulated) practices. Milk banks are portrayed as saving lives (Carroll, 2014); milk sharing as risking lives (Carter et al., 2015). Cross-nursing (breastfeeding someone else's baby) engenders strong feelings in others – the 'yuk' (Shaw, 2004) or 'ick' (Vogel, 2011) factor, also often seen in relation to breastfeeding that is perceived to go on 'too long' (Dowling and Brown, 2013).

These ways of thinking about breastmilk inevitably also influence how it is thought about in relation to donation. The history and process of managing milk donated to milk banks is one of medicalisation and dehumanisation (Swanson, 2014) and this can be seen, in part, as attempting to remove negative associations with women's bodily fluids. Donated milk (expressed from a woman's breasts) becomes a product in a milk bank, labelled as PDHM (pasteurised donor human milk) or BDM (banked donor milk) and is removed from associations with the body it came from. There is evidence that for some women (donating or receiving breastmilk for their baby), this depersonalisation is helpful, as they prefer not to think about the milk as coming from another mother or going to another's baby (Zizzo, 2011). Some would happily donate to a milk bank but feel uneasy about cross-nursing (Shaw, 2010) while for others the personal connection is the motivation for informal milk sharing (Gribble, 2013).

Ways of thinking about breastmilk sharing and donation

Waldby (2015a) has noted that body tissues are being used in new and unprecedented ways; breastmilk too is being used in ways that are both old and new. It can be argued that breastmilk donation is fundamentally different to other forms of donation, such as blood, eggs or organs, although Waldby has also noted there is also an unregulated market in other human tissues, perhaps especially:

> for tissues considered non-essential to the life of the donor ...
>
> (2015b, p. 275)

She cites the example of hair, but also eggs (ooctytes). Breastmilk is primarily formed in the body of a lactating body in order to go into the
body of another human being (her child), although interestingly, when
used in this way, breastmilk is not seen as 'donation' and only when used
to feed another child does the terminology change (Kent et al., 2017).
The increased availability and use of breast pumps and ease of storage means that breastmilk can leave a lactating body and travel in new
ways, as a *'mobile biosubstance'* (Boyer, 2010). Unlike other bodily fluids
and organs (with perhaps the exception of semen), it can be exchanged
easily, informally and for free. There are also, perhaps unlike other forms
of donation, strong cultural meanings associated with breastmilk. These
are both those relating to the ways in which women's bodies are seen
and understood (as discussed above) and to specific cultural beliefs, for
example in relation to milk kinship in Islam. People are considered to be
related to each other if they have both received breastmilk from the same
woman and therefore prohibited from, for example marriage with each
other – this latter example has led to particular challenges for milk banking (UKAMB, 2017c).

A number of issues have been considered in the literature in relation to
breastmilk sharing, although, as with much of the work in this area, this
is usually focused around US law and thinking, as these have not been
formally considered in other countries. This is complicated by the fact
that there is some exchange of breastmilk for money as well as the ways
in which it has been written about (primarily conceived as a gift). Shaw,
writing about informed consent and cross-nursing (when women know or
have met one another, although the issues may be similar for women who
have never met), cites Gilligan (1982) and Vaughan (2004) and notes that

> women's actions are often determined in relation to the needs and interests of
> others, not simply in terms of abstract principles of give and take ...
>
> (2007, p. 439)

It might not, therefore, be quite as straightforward as in other examples
to think about this form of donation simply in terms of a gift relationship
(after Titmuss, 1970) or a commercial exchange. Ideas of reciprocity are
important in Shaw's example of women who breastfeed one another's
babies, although this may be less important in internet relationships,
where the milk is likely to only be given or received and not exchanged.

Although the focus of this chapter is on the exchange or sharing of
breastmilk, in the literature the issues about sharing and selling are often
conflated and so I discuss both here. Where there are laws, such as those
in many countries regarding the selling of bodily materials, both the sale
and exchange of breastmilk and breastmilk could be seen in this way.

Likewise, selling adulterated products (e.g. watered-down breastmilk) can be an offence, as would be knowingly transmitting a communicable disease (Dawson David, 2011). Regulating how women use their bodies and bodily products would, however, be seen by many as unacceptable; it can be argued that breasts, breastmilk and breastfeeding are personal and not community property (Schmidt, 2008). Breastmilk is considered a human tissue under UK Human Tissue Authority regulations and is in the list of materials considered to be 'relevant material' under the Human Tissue Act 2004 (HTA, 2014a); this has some relevance to how it is stored and used. Breastmilk for human consumption, however, is not listed as 'Material covered by the Quality and Safety for Human Application Regulations 2007' (HTA, 2014b).

Issues for health professionals and volunteer supporters

Why do the issues in this chapter matter? Are these not private issues, which should fall outside of the scope of regulation or professional practice? Even if we argue, as I do, that this is so, there are still ways in which health professionals might need to be aware of, and consider responses to, questions that may be asked of them in relation to informal milk sharing, or obtaining breastmilk via the internet. In the United States, the American Academy of Nursing on Policy have published a 'Position Statement' for health professionals (2016); to date nothing similar exists for UK nurses and midwives. In the UK, health professionals may be asked for advice; responses may be influenced by lack of knowledge but also by personal opinion (perhaps by the 'yuk factor', discussed above). They may also be shaped by strongly worded reporting (Steele et al., 2015a) and a call for action, for example:

> Health professionals and regulators both must be aware of this growing trend and issue public guidance against the purchasing of human milk from Internet sources for adult as well as infant feeding ...
>
> (Steele et al., 2015a)

How do healthcare professionals make judgements about this and know what to say to pregnant or lactating women? How can they understand the issues, especially when much of the writing about this conflates the issues (and risks) relating to buying and selling, donating and receiving freely given milk?

Nurses and midwives have a responsibility to provide evidence-based care and advice (NMC, 2015). However, there is a lack of clear information for both health professionals and mothers, and the onus is on women to protect themselves and their children. This relies, to a large extent, on truth-telling and trust – and so what is the health professional's role in this? Do we need to think about clearer advice to give to women who want to share breastmilk – or is it a private matter? What would be the position of the health professional should a baby subsequently become unwell? Do we need regulation? What would be a good source of information for health professionals on risks – and how do we make judgements about these? Evidence-based information on how to share milk safely – such as that provided by breastmilk sharing organisations via their websites might be a good starting point (see 'The four pillars of safe breastmilk sharing', Eats on Feets, 2017). Although not bound in the same way by regulatory bodies, those working for voluntary organisations (such as La Leche League [LLL], NCT [National Childbirth Trust], Association of Breastfeeding Mothers [ABM], The Breastfeeding Network [BFN]) may face similar dilemmas and need to consider their approach and position.

Conclusion

Donating breastmilk has increased, particularly in informal relationships facilitated by the internet and social media, although how much this is happening in the UK is unknown. In some countries, ideas of risk frame the 'official' reaction to sharing breastmilk via the internet, although there is no guidance in the UK. Research, mainly from the United States, informs a growing understanding of the issues, although little is known about how women in the UK understand and make sense of any potential risks. Donating and receiving breastmilk has arisen in woman-to-woman grassroots ways, in a similar way to other forms of breastfeeding support, and these can be seen as acts of care. Although there are some common issues, breastmilk donation differs from other forms of donation in important ways – and raises some specific ethical dilemmas for healthcare workers and others.

References

Akre, J.E., Gribble, K.D. and Minchin, M. (2011) Milk sharing: from private practice to public pursuit. *International Breastfeeding Journal*, 6(1), p. 8.

American Academy of Nursing on Policy (2016) Position statement regarding use of informatlly shared human milk. *Nursing Outlook*, 64(1), pp. 98–102.

Boyer, K. (2010) Of care and commodities: breastmilk and the new politics of mobile biosubstances. *Progress in Human Geography*, 34(5), pp. 5–20.

Boyer, K. (2014) 'Neoliberal motherhood': workplace lactation and changing conceptions of working motherhood in the contemporary US. *Feminist Theory*, 15(3), pp. 269–88.

Carroll, K. (2014) Body dirt or liquid gold? How the 'safety' of donated breastmilk is constructed for use in neonatal intensive care. *Social Studies of Science*, 44(3), pp. 466–85.

Carroll, K. (2015) Breastmilk donation as care work. In Cassidy, T. and El Tom, A. (eds), *Ethnographies of Breastfeeding* (pp. 173–86). London/New Delhi/New York/Sidney: Bloomsbury.

Carter, S.K., Reyes-Foster, B. and Rogers, T.L. (2015) Liquid gold or Russian roulette?: Risk and human milk sharing in the U.S. news media. *Health, Risk and Society*, 17(1), pp. 30–45.

Carter, S.K. and Reyes-Foster, B.M. (2016) Pure gold for broken bodies: discursive techniques constructing milk banking and peer milk sharing in U.S. news. *Symbolic Interaction*, 39(3), pp. 353–73.

Cassidy, T. (2012) Making 'milky matches': globalization, maternal trust and 'lactivist' online networking. *Journal of the Motherhood Initiative*, (3)2, pp. 226–40.

Cohen, R.S., Xiong, S.C. and Sakamoto, P. (2009) Retrospective review of serological testing of potential human milk donors. *Archives Diseases in Childhood Fetal Neonatal Edition*, 95(2), pp. F118–20, DOI: 10.1136/adc.2008.15647.

Dawson David, S. (2011) Legal commentary on the sale of human milk. *Public Health Reports*, 126(2), pp. 165–166.

Douglas, M. ([1966] 2002) *Purity and Danger*. London/New York: Routledge.

Dowling, S. and Brown, A. (2013) An exploration of the experiences of mothers who breastfeed long-term: what are the issues and why does it matter? *Breastfeeding Medicine*, 8(1), pp. 45–52, DOI: 10.1089/bfm.2012.0057.

Dowling, S., Naidoo, J. and Pontin, D. (2012) Breastfeeding in public: women's bodies, women's milk. In P. Smith, H.B. Hall and M. Labbok (eds), *Beyond Health, Beyond Choice: Breastfeeding Constraints and Realities* (pp. 249–58). New Brunswick/New Jersey: Rutgers University Press.

Dowling, S. and Pontin, D. (2017) Using liminality to understand mothers' experiences of long-term breastfeeding: 'betwixt and between', and 'matter out of place'. *Health: An Interdisciplinary Journal for the Social Study of Health, Illness and Medicine,* 21(1), pp. 57–75.

Eats on Feets. (2017) The four pillars of safe breast milk sharing. http://www.eatsonfeets.org/#fourPillars (accessed 25 January 2018).

Geraghty, S., Khoury, J. and Kalkwarf, H. (2005) Human milk pumping rates of mothers of singletons and mothers of multiples. *Journal of Human Lactation*, 21(4), pp. 413–20.

Geraghty, S.R., Heier, J.E. and Rasmussen, K.M. (2011) Got milk? Sharing human milk via the internet. *Public Health Reports*, 126(2), pp. 161–64.

Gilligan, C. (1982, 1993) *In a different voice*. Harvard: Harvard University Press

Gribble, K. (2013) Peer-to-peer milk donors' and recipients' experiences of donor milk banks. *Journal of Obstetric, Gynecologic, & Neonatal Nursing*, 42(4), pp. 451–61.

Gribble, K. and Hausman, B.L. (2012) Milk sharing and formula feeding: infant feeding risks in comparative perspective? *Australasian Medical Journal*, 5(5), pp. 275–83.

Hausman, B.L. (2004) The feminist politics of breastfeeding. *Australian Feminist Studies*, 19(45), pp. 273–85.

Hausman, B. (2011) *Viral Bodies: Breastfeeding in the Age of HIV/AIDS*. Ann Arbor, MI: University of Michigan Press.

Keim, S.A., McNamara, K.A., Jayadeva, C.M. et al. (2014) Breast milk sharing via the internet: the practice and health and safety considerations. *Maternal and Child Health Journal*, 18(6), pp. 1471–79.

Keim, A.A., Hogan, J.S. and McNamara, C.A. (2013) Microbial contamination of human milk purchased via the internet. *Pediatrics*, 132(5), pp. e1227–35.

Kent, J., Fannin, M. and Dowling, S. (2017) Gender dynamics in the donation field: human tissue donation for research, therapy and feeding. In *Royal Geographical Society (with IBG)*, London, England, 29 August–1 September 2017. http://eprints.uwe.ac.uk/33006.

La Leche League GB (2017) Sharing breastmilk. https://www.laleche.org.uk/sharing-breastmilk/ (accessed 25 January 2018).

McFadden, A., Gavine, A., Renfrew, M.J., Wade, A., Buchanan, P., Taylor, J.L., Veitch, E., et al. (2017) *Support for healthy breastfeeding mothers with healthy term babies*. Cochrane Database of Systematic Reviews 2017, 2. Art. No.: CD001141, DOI: 10.1002/14651858.CD001141.pub5.

Nursing & Midwifery Council (NMC). (2015) *The code for nurses and midwives*. https://www.nmc.org.uk/standards/code/ (accessed 25 January 2018).

NICE (2010) Donor milk banks: the operation of donor milk bank services (NICE clinical guideline 93). http://www.nice.org.uk/guidance/cg93/resources/guidance-donor-milk-banks-the-operation-of-donor-milk-bank-services-pdf (accessed 25 January 2018).

Only the Breast (2017) *Post an ad and help babies get Only The Breast*. http://www.onlythebreast.com (accessed 25 January 2018).

Palmer, G. (2009) *The Politics of Breastfeeding: When Breasts Are Bad for Business*. London: Pinter and Martin.

Palmquist, A. (2015) Demedicalizing breastmilk: the discourses, practices and identities of informal milk sharing. In T. Cassidy and A. El Tom (eds), *Ethnographies of Breastfeeding* (pp. 23–44). London/New Delhi/New York/Sidney: Bloomsbury.

Palmquist, A.E.L. and Doehler, K. (2014) Contextualizing online human milk sharing: structural factors and lactation disparity among middle income women in the U.S. *Social Science and Medicine*, 122, pp. 140–47.

Palmquist, A.E.L. and Doehler, K. (2015) Human milk sharing practices in the U.S. *Maternal and Child Nutrition*, 12(2), pp. 278–90.

Pokhrel, S., Quigley, M.A., Fox-Rushby, J., McCormick, F., Williams, A., Trueman, P., Dodds, R. et al. (2015) Potential economic impacts from improving breastfeeding rates in the UK. *Archives Disease Child*, 100, pp. 334–40, DOI: 10.1136/archdischild-2014-306701.

Rollins, N.C., Bhandari, N., Hajeebhoy, N. et al. (2016) Why invest, and what it will take to improve breastfeeding practices? *Lancet*, 387(10017), pp. 491–504, DOI: http://dx.doi.org/10.1016/S0140-6736(15)01044-2.

Shaw, R. (2004) The virtues of cross-nursing and the 'yuk factor'. *Australian Feminist Studies*, 19(45), pp. 287–99.

Shaw, R. (2007) Cross-nursing, ethics, and giving breastmilk in the contemporary context. *Women's Studies International Forum*, 30(5), pp. 439–50.

Schmidt, J. (2008) Gendering in infant feeding discourses: the good mother and the absent father. *New Zealand Sociology*, 23(2), pp. 61–74.

Stearns, C. (2010) The breast pump. In R. Shaw and A. Bartlett (eds), *Giving Breast Milk: Body Ethics and Contemporary Practice* (pp. 11–23). Toronto: Demeter Press.

Steele, S., Martyn, J. and Foell, J. (2015a) Risks of the unregulated market in human breastmilk: Urgent need for regulation. *British Medical Journal*, 350, p. h1485, DOI: 10.1136/bmj.h1485.

Steele, S., Foell, J., Martyn, J. and Freitag, A. (2015b) More than a lucrative liquid: the risks for adult consumers of human breast milk bought from the online market. *Journal of the Royal Society of Medicine*, 108(6), pp. 208–9, DOI: 10.1177/0141076815588539.

Swanson, K.W. (2014) *Banking on the Body: The Market in Blood, Milk and Sperm in Modern America*. Cambridge, MA, and London: Harvard University Press.

Titmuss, R.M. (1970) *The Gift Relationship: From Human Blood to Social Policy*. London: George Allen and Unwin.

United Kingdom Association of Milk Banking (2016a) *Speaking to potential donors*. http://www.ukamb.org/speaking-potential-donors/ (accessed 25 January 2018).

United Kingdom Association of Milk Banking (2016b) *Breastmilk sharing – a statement from UKAMB*. http://www.ukamb.org/breastmilk-sharing-statement-ukamb/ (accessed 25 January 2018).

UKAMB (2017c) *Resolution on the Use of Donor Human Milk for Muslim Infants*. http://www.ukamb.org/resolution-use-donor-human-milk-muslim-infants/ (accessed 25 January 2018).

UK Human Tissue Authority (2014a) *List of materials considered to be 'relevant material' under the Human Tissue Act 2004*. https://www.hta.gov.uk/policies/list-materials-considered-be-'relevant-material'-under-human-tissue-act-2004 (accessed 25 January 2018).

UK Human Tissue Authority (2014b) *Material covered by the Quality and Safety for Human Application Regulations 2007*. https://www.hta.gov.uk/policies/material-covered-quality-and-safety-human-application-regulations (accessed 25 January 2018).

UNICEF UK (2016) Protecting health and saving lives: a call to action. https://www.unicef.org.uk/babyfriendly/baby-friendly-resources/advocacy/call-to-action/ (accessed 25 January 2018).

Vaughan, G. (2004), *The gift, il dono: a feminist analysis*. Rome: Meltemi editore

Victora, C.G., Bahl, R., Barros, A.J.D. et al (2016). Breastfeeding in the 21st century: epidemiology, mechanisms, and lifelong effect. *Lancet*, 387(10017), pp. 475–90.

Vogel, L. (2011) Milk sharing: or biohazard? *Canadian Medical Association Journal*, 183(3), E155–56, DOI: 10.1503/cmaj.109-3767

Waldby, C. (2015a) 'Banking time': freezing and the negotiation of future fertility. *Culture, Health and Sexuality*, 17(4), pp. 470–82.

Waldby, C. (2015b) The oocyte market and social egg freezing: scarcity to singularity. *Journal of Cultural Economy*, 8(3), pp. 275–91

Welborn, J.M. (2012) The experience of expressing and donating breastmilk following a perinatal loss. *Journal of Human Lactation*, 28(4), pp. 506–10.

West, E. and Knight, R. J. (2017) Mothers' milk: Slavery, wet-nursing, and black and white women in the antebellum South. *Journal of Southern History, The Southern Historical Association*, 83(1), pp. 37–68.

WHO/UNICEF (2003) *Global Strategy for Infant and Young Child Feeding*. Geneva: World Health Organisation.

Zizzo, G. (2011) 'Donor breastmilk is a product from the hospital, not somebody': dissassociation in contemporary milk banking. *Outskirts Online Journal*, 24.

6

Veterans and the ethics of reciprocity

Hilary Engward

Introduction

In the UK, The Armed Forces Covenant is a promise from the nation that those who have served in the Armed Forces and are injured from that service should receive priority treatment in the National Health Service (NHS), where a condition results from their service, subject to clinical need (Ministry of Defence, 2011). Increasing numbers of soldiers living with long-term injuries raises questions about the nature of the provision of medical care for veterans with long-term and chronic health conditions. The purpose of this chapter is to explore the nature of the entitlement to prioritised care in relation to veterans. As most health service practitioners will at some point care for veterans, decisions about if and how a veteran ought to be prioritised need to be articulated, including questions as to whether veterans are distinctly vulnerable from other groups in society and if so, how their needs can be ethically balanced against those of other vulnerable groups.

Who are veterans?

In the UK, the legal term *veteran* encompasses anyone who has served for at least one day in the Armed Forces (regular or reserve) in uniform. In the UK, the Armed Forces community of serving personnel, reservists, their families and veterans is approximately 10 million people, of which roughly 2.8 million are Armed Forces veterans (NHS, 2015). The largest age band of UK veterans is 65+ years, approximately 28 per cent of the overall 65+ years UK population (Age UK, 2015). From recent wars (Iraq and Afghanistan), greater numbers of casualties survived battlefield injuries, with younger injured veterans more likely to live longer than previously due to enhanced body armour and medical evacuation (Fossey and Hacker Hughes, 2014); many have severe injuries to areas not directly protected by body armour, such as the head and neck. The nature of the military experience has also changed over time, with the term *new wars* being used to characterise the nature of possible harm that deployment might incur, such as bearing witness to atrocities such as child soldiers, civilian population expulsion, exemplary violence, torture and sexual assault (Castles and Miller, 1998)

The armed forces covenant

The concept of a covenant in relation to the Armed Forces was first codified in a paragraph in *Soldiering: The Military Covenant* (2000) and at its simplest presented an understanding that in exchange for their service and sacrifice, soldiers will be supported by their nation and chain of command. It is likely that the concept would have gained little traction in the public sphere if it hadn't been for interventions in Iraq and Afghanistan. Seen as wars of choice rather than necessity by the public, the then Labour Government sought to convince a sceptical public that such intervention was inevitable, and during electioneering in 2010, the Covenant was used to focus on the welfare of the Armed Forces. In 2011, the Armed Forces Covenant was introduced by the then Coalition government and gave statutory recognition to the concept. The Armed Forces Covenant is integral in British Defence Policy and has provided a new lens through which we can view the civil-military relationship.

The Armed Forces Covenant as it currently stands encapsulates fundamental principles which apply to all service personnel, veterans and their families, who share, or have shared, a commitment to serve the nation, including the suspension of their personal liberties and unlimited liability, from which it is appropriate to persume a mutual expectation of how they should be treated by government and society in return. By definition, a covenant is a contract, which suggests that the forces and government could generalise their respective responsibilities, with legal sanction available when the contract is breached. In fact, there is no legal guarantee or basis in UK law, custom or history for the Covenant, and the Armed Forces Act itself guarantees no such Covenant. This coupled with the very nature of the military, with its innate unpredictability of circumstances, makes the activation of such a contract troublesome, and as always, cases are formed within a historical legacy and what is currently the situation. For example, some accommodation service personnel are assigned to remains poor; however, service personnel have little choice other than to accept it as they cannot decline posting on the basis of standards of housing. The Covenant is, as such, a living document that brings to light how current circumstance is historically situated, for example how individual services chose to allocate insufficient funding to maintaining the estate from their budget allocations, which is set within a historical legacy as to how that resourcing has occurred (the Ministry of Defence [MOD] resolves to continue improvement to service personel accomodation, 2008). However, what the Covenant does is bring to the fore questions as to how we ought to respect and treat persons in the Armed Forces, veterans and their families. In other words, what do we, as a society, owe to our service and ex-service personnel in return for their allegiance to keeping our nation safe? The ethics of reciprocity goes some way to helping us understand this relationship better, and for the purpose of this chapter, it is viewed in relation to accessing health and medical care, although it could be equally applied in relation to gaining housing and employment.

The ethics of reciprocity and veterans

Ethically, reciprocity refers to the mutual exchange of privileges from one party to another, with the aim of establishing and maintaining equality between the parties. In relation to veterans, the concept of reciprocity refers to society's recognition of prior service in the Armed Forces that will in turn be rewarded with prioritised health service access and treatment for health conditions directly associated with that service. In the UK, therefore, all veterans are entitled to priority access to NHS hospital care for any condition so long as it is related to their service, and subject to the clinical need of others, as set out in The Armed Forces Covenant, which, in turn, outlines the relationship between the nation, the government and the Armed Forces.

It may seem odd that the nature of what ought to be owed to veterans in relation to healthcare has not received more attention in the literature, and this discrepancy likely lies in the difference between military and civilian medicine. The purpose of military medicine is to care for those who can fight, rather than saving the lives of those who cannot, and military medical ethics is guided by a principle of military necessity and 'salvage,' that is, to return soldiers to duty. Soldiers who cannot return to battle fall under the non-military or civilian medicine, which is governed by the laws of medical need and focuses its efforts on saving lives and maintaining quality of life. This means that when soldiers are fit to fight, military medicine will devote resources to maintaining their health so they may continue to serve national interests. However, once unable to return to duty, soldiers become patients, and the principle of medical need that governs their care is blind to their former military identity. Once service personnel cannot return to duty, they lose their unique entitlement to military medical resources and thus compete equally with similarly injured and sick civilians for care. Paradoxically, therefore, it is assumed that the best way to care for injured service persons may be to disregard their status as soldiers and focus on their status as patients. It is in this sense that in some countries, such as the UK, military hospitals have mostly closed, and the distinction between military and civilian medicine is an anachronism.

The moral justifications for privileged care are difficult to articulate, and although those seriously wounded in battle surely deserve something, there is room to ask whether they deserve something better than everyone else does. McCartney (2009) states that there will always be a gap between what service personnel want and what the public might be willing to give, and questions remain as to how much the UK is willing to care for its veterans in line with other competing health needs, and what it is ethical to provide. The following section teases apart argument as to if and why there ought to be a case for priority access to healthcare for veterans in the UK context.

The case for priority access to health service

In the UK, the NHS provides the right for healthcare that all citizens can access; in general, special interest groups do not gain special entitlements, but rather gain healthcare commensurate with that which is best available. One exception to this rule is for conditions related to military service, where the Department of Health directs that veterans, at their first outpatient appointment, ought to be 'scheduled for treatment quicker than other patients of similar clinical priority'.

The central ethical question, therefore, is what makes a veteran more worthy, or unique, to gain prioritised access to health services in relation to other groups. One such criterion is the distinctive nature of the military culture. Military personnel are socialised, through basic training, to adhere to military cultural norms of acceptance of regimentation, hierarchy and depersonalisation in favour of the collective, and it is this very specific view of the social world that radically differs from the civilian social world. For some veterans, the move from active military service to civilian life is a major change in culture, leading to problems in independently gaining housing and employment, and adjusting to civilian cultural norms (Cooper et al., 2016). Cohn (1999) defines this as a 'cultural gap' in which differences in the norms, values and culture between the military and civilian spheres exists, leading to a 'connectivity gap' and diminishing contact between the Armed Forces and society. In relation to the UK, Cohn concludes that these lead to a 'respect–value' gap, characterised by citizens respecting but placing little value on the sacrifice of those placed in harm's way to serve the state. The Armed Forces Covenant goes some way to address any respect–value gap by stating what military and veterans and their families are entitled to expect from health services. For example, for those with 'concerns about their mental health, where symptoms may not present for some time after leaving Service, they should be able to access services with health professionals who have an understanding of the Armed Forces culture'. Whether this actually occurs is debatable. This in turn may be problematic to health professionals, as it is unclear as to how much of an understanding healthcare professionals and workers have about the nature of military experience.

It also cannot be assumed that veterans will have health needs that differ from the civilian population, and not all health problems are directly attributable to military service; for example, only 50 per cent of post-traumatic stress disorder (PTSD) cases in currently serving personnel can be directly attributed to deployment. Rather, it should be recognised that any potential vulnerability that results from being or having been in military service is unique and distinct from the civilian population, and it is this potential vulnerability that creates a distinct ethical duty to prioritise care for this group. This indeed could be where the overarching uniqueness for the ethic of reciprocity lies, but the extent to how this is played out in contemporary healthcare provision for veterans needs further inquiry and understanding (Forster, 2012).

Another criterion to prioritised access is access based on individual medical need, and at face value it seems reasonable to suggest that access to services can be based on objective clinical judgement. The problem with this argument is that medical need in itself is not neutral, but rather confers values as to what is more important. Prolongation of life, elimination of disease, and improved quality of life, are all important health needs, but how these are to be ranked in relation to one another, if at all, is unclear. For example, if a prior established health need that has been attributed to previous military service is exacerbated by the current socio-economic living conditions of the veteran, this could be as equally experienced by other members of that community. Possibly from popularised media reporting, there is an assumption that the veteran population in the UK are vulnerable to mental health issues, higher rates of homelessness, alcohol misuse, domestic violence, relationship breakdown and criminal activity (Woodhead et al., 2007). This may be the case, but it could be conversely argued that any persons who experience change in employment and/or living conditions are equally susceptible to such health concerns.

If the veteran's level of need is the same as that of other members of the general public, but the veteran is given priority, then 'need' cannot be the only rationale for the veteran's priority, and all other things being equal, priority again must stem from the veteran's status as a veteran. Veterans, in other words, merit care in a way that non-veterans do not, because of the service they have provided to the nation. There is some evidence of public support for this idea; for example, the UK public showed support for British citizenship rights for retired Ghurkas, with a notion that something was owed to the soldiers in return for the risks they were exposed to on the UK's behalf (The Guardian, 2016). This refers to reciprocity as demanding that those who have been exposed to exceptional risks be entitled to commensurate consideration. However, others also place themselves in danger in order to serve the nation, for example firefighters, paramedics and the police, who are not afforded prioritised access to healthcare if injury results from service. Rather, it is the distinctive uniqueness of the suspension of personal liberties and unlimited liability for the good of the nation as a whole that is the difference between the military and other public service professions.

It therefore seems reasonable to assume that those who place themselves in exceptional potential danger to protect our national interests ought to be rewarded in kind. If this is the case, how extensive is this obligation? The question here is about the nature, or origin, of the injury. For example, service personnel may be injured because they were placed in undue circumstances of risk, but not all service personnel will have been active in the front-line theatre of war. For example, should those who work in information technology, far from the front line, be entitled to the same prioritised medical care? If two service personnel have the same injury, one in a car accident at home on leave, and another as a result of combat in war, should both, as veterans, have equal access to accelerated health services as a result of that injury while in service? What if injury results from a deliberate choice not to follow procedure? For example, some head injuries from Vietnam occurred when soldiers did not wear helmets because they were too hot and uncomfortable (Neel, 1991). Similarly in Iraq, some soldiers did not wear goggles (Gwanda, 2004), so are head and eye injuries resulting from a personal choice not to wear protective clothing less worthy of care? The answer to all these questions may be that, as healthcare is a basic human right, we cannot distinguish based either on circumstance or behavioural choices, and treatment must always be given according to medical need alone. A comparison here, for example, is for those who choose to engage in dangerous recreational activity, such as rock climbing, to receive medical care as based on the nature of the injury rather than due to the activity itself. If this is the case, then military service should not add to, or detract from, an individual's right to healthcare; rather, the person has the right to access healthcare based on that injury alone.

There is also another dimension to this debate. Over the last decade, increasing numbers of active service personnel, veterans and families of those killed at war have questioned whether inadequate resources put soldiers at unnecessary risk. With possibilities of depleted resources following a 15 per cent reduction in defence spending (Royal United Services Institute, 2010), there is a risk that serving personnel may knowingly be at increased risk of harm and injury. On the one hand, therefore, the covenant provides the soldier with a clause of unlimited liability, and on the other, places the worth of equipment beyond the scope of this protection. This suggests that concepts within the Covenant are flexible or, in the at least, subject to political interpretation.

If, however, we accept that veterans are unique, then ought veterans to have access to veteran-specific health services? While there are examples of veteran-specific service provision in the UK, for example, there are ring-fenced monies within the NHS budget for veteran mental healthcare; most specific healthcare provision is limited to prosthetic services. There has also been an increase of new third-sector providers alongside established brands such as the Royal British Legion and Combat Stress, which deliver veteran-specific care and support; for example, Blesma, The Limbless Veterans, offers support for those with limb loss and loss of use. This has resulted in different approaches, interventions, post-code patterns of delivery and a difference in governance procedures. It is also unclear as to where the boundaries of treatment versus support for the individual/ families lie. This also assumes that veterans may prefer to see clinicians with an understanding of and sensitivity towards military life and culture (Ben-Zeev et al., 2012), and while 'veteran-informed' or 'veteran-specific' services may be relevant to some individuals, there are likely to be others who would not want either (Greenberg et al., 2003). Indeed, helping veterans manage health and well-being concerns is important given the demands placed on military personnel (Ministry of Defence, 2015), but to date, the nature of the veteran in the health sector is poorly understood and there is minimal research that explores the nature of this experience.

Conclusion

This chapter has sought to increase awareness of the veteran in the health sector, and to raise important questions about the nature and scope of the State's duty to care for veterans. The Armed Forces Covenant tells us that where veterans receive healthcare in the NHS, care should be prioritised where the condition is a result of their service in the Armed Forces.

This chapter has argued that, due to the unique nature of being in the military, prioritised access can be justifiable, but only when that injury can be directly attributable to that service. It is not easy to determine if symptoms are directly related to that service, and when this is questioned, treatment ought to be based on clinical need alone. Past military contribution therefore does not necessarily always confer prioritised access to health services, but may rather operate as a 'tie breaker' when there are many patients of equal need. Prioritised access to services for veterans may be ethically defensible when the services required are related to the injuries during military service *and* only when no other patient with more urgent medical needs requires attention.

References

Age UK. (2015) Later life in the United Kingdom. http://www.ageuk.org.uk/Documents/ENGB/Factsheets/Later_Life_UK_factsheet.pdf?dtrk=true.

Ben-Zeev, D., Corrigan, P.W., Britt, T.W. and Langford, L. (2012) Stigma of mental illness and service use in the military. *Journal of Mental Health*, 21(3), pp. 264–73.

Cohn, L. (1999). The evolution of the civil-military 'gap' debate. Paper prepared for the TISS project on the gap between the military and civil society. http://static1.1.sqspcdn.com/static/f/1472877/18563652/1338821276343/Cohn_Evolution+of+Gap+Debate+1999.pdf?token=yZEfMzwHIVYqSky27I2j18aSA6A%3D.

Cooper, L., Andrews, S. and Fossey, M. (2016). Educating nurses to care for military veterans in civilian hospitals: An integrative literature review. *Nursing Education Today*, 47, pp. 68–73.

Castles, S. and Miller, M.J. (1998) *The Age of Migration: International Population Movements in the Modern World*, 2nd edn. New York: Guilford Press.

Fossey, M. and Hacker Hughes, J. (2014) *Traumatic Limb Loss and the Needs of the Family: Current Research: Policy and Practice Implications*. London: Blesma.

Forster, A. (2012). The military covenant and British military-civilian relations: Letting the genie out of the bottle. *Armed Forces and Society*, 38(2), pp. 273–90.

Greenberg, N., Thomas, S., Iversen, A., Unwin, C., Hull, L. and Wessely, S. (2003) Do military peacekeepers want to talk about their experiences? Perceived psychological support of UK military peacekeepers on return from deployment. *Journal of Mental Health*, 12(6), pp. 565–73.

Gwanda, A. (2004) Casualties of war – military care for the wounded from Iraq and Aghanistan. *New England Journal of Medicine*, 251, pp. 2471–75.

McCartney, H. (2009). The Military Covenant and the changing civilian-military contract in Britain. Paper presented at the Inter-University Armed Forces seminar, Chicago, October 24, 11.

Ministry of Defence (2011) The Armed Forces Covenant: Today and Tomorrow. https://www.gov.uk/government/uploads/system/uploads/attachment_data/

file/49470/the_armed_forces_covenant_today_and_tomorrow.pdf (accessed 30 October 2015).

Ministry of Defence. (2015) Armed Forces Covenant. May. www.gov.uk/ government/policies/fulfilling-the-commitments-of-the-armed-forces-covenant/supporting-pages/armed-forces-community-covenant (accessed 14 October 2015).

Neel, S. (1991). *Medical support of the US army in Vietnam 1965–1970*. Washington, DC: US Department of the Army, p. 55.

National Health Services Choices (2015) NHS healthcare for veterans. http:// www.nhs.uk/NHSEngland/Militaryhealthcare/veterans-families-reservists/ Pages/veterans.aspx (accessed 14 October 2015).

Royal United Services Institute. (2010) Prognosis for defence spending after Budget 2010. https://rusi.org/commentary/prognosis-defence-spending-after-budget-2010.

The Guardian. (2016) Gurkha veterans claim victory in court battle for UK visas. https://www.theguardian.com/uk/2008/sep/30/military.immigration (accessed 1 August 2016).

Woodhead, C., Rona, R.J., Iveron, A., McManus, D., Hotopf, M., Dean, K., et al. (2007) Mental health and health service use among post national service veterans: Results from the 2007 Adult Psychiatric Morbidity Survey in England. *Psychological Medicine*, 41(2), pp. 363–72.

7

In whose best interests?

Zoe Picton-Howell

Best interests

Paediatricians in the United Kingdom (UK) are guided by their rules of professional conduct (General Medical Council, 2013) to ensure that all decisions made on behalf of children (including young people) (General Medical Council, 2013a) under the age of 16[1] are made in the child's 'best interests'.

'Best interests of the child' is a well-established concept in international and domestic law. Article 3 of the *United Nations Convention on the Rights of Child* states 'In all actions concerning children ... the best interest of the child shall be a primary consideration.'[2] The best interests of the child have been described as the 'golden thread', which runs 'throughout the tangled web of English family law'.[3] The 'welfare of the child', a phrase often used synonymously with 'best interests', is paramount in English and Scottish Law.[4] The phrase 'best interests' is mentioned in some 208 pieces of UK legislation[5] And the English Courts have analysed what 'best interests' means in healthcare over the last 45 years, making clear best interests must be considered

---

[1] Once a young person reaches the age of 16, the Mental Capacity Act 2005 c.9 applies.

[2] Article 3, Paragraph 1, Convention of the Rights of the Child, adopted and opened for signature, ratification and accession by United Nations General Assembly resolution 44/25 of 20 November 1989. Entry into force 2 September 1990, in accordance with article 49, ratified by United Kingdom on 16 December 1991 and came into force on 15 January 1992.

[3] Lord St. John of Fawsley (2007) *'House of Lords Debate'*, Hansard, 31 January, C227.

[4] s. 1 (1) Children Act 1989 (c.41); s.16 (1) Children (Scotland) Act 1995.

[5] 208 pieces of legislation from the UK are listed in the British and Irish Legal Information Institute's database of UK legislation as containing the phrase *best interests*, http://www.bailii.org.

in the widest sense, taking into account, where appropriate, a wide range of ethical, social, moral, emotional and welfare considerations. (Burke, 2004, per Munby).[6]

Although the primacy of a child's best interests in law is clear, different understandings of the relevant facts and different values from those involved can lead to disagreements as to what is in an individual child's best interests (Larcher et al., 2015: 10, para 2.2.1). These disagreements can have important ethical implications not just for the children but also for their parents and the doctors involved.

Disagreement

The disagreements as to infant Charlie Gard's[7] best interests made headline news nationally and internationally during the first six months of 2017. Charlie's story hit the headlines just as I was writing up research on UK paediatricians' best interests decision-making for severely disabled children. My research included surveys and semi-structured interviews with a small group of UK paediatricians and discussion of disagreements featured prominently. Drawing on some of the findings from that research, together with wider literature reviews of parents' experiences of end-of-life discussions with doctors, this chapter explores the everyday disagreements that can arise when end-of-life best interests decisions are being made for severely disabled children. It will also consider whether the ethical guidance provided to paediatricians by their professional bodies helps or hinders the resolution of these disagreements and explore some of the ethical implications these disagreements pose, not just for the children at the centre of the decisions but also for their parents and the doctors.

The children

The children the doctors in my study discussed can be distinguished from Charlie Gard, and indeed most of the children whose cases have

---

[6] *Burke, R (on the application of) vs The General Medical Council*, Rev 1 [2004] EWHC 1879 (Admin) (30 July 2004); per Munby, para. 90.
[7] *Great Ormond Street Hospital v. Yates & Gard* [2017]EWHC 972 (Fam); *Yates & Anor vs Great Ormond Street Hospital for Children NHS Foundation Trust & Anor* (Rev 1) [2017] EWCA Civ 410 (23 May 2017) Gard (A Child), Re [2017] EWHC 1909 (Fam) (24 July 2017); *Gard and Others vs the United Kingdom* – 39793/17 (Decision [2017] ECHR 605 (27 June 2017).

come before the English courts,[8] in a number of ways. The children have lived beyond infancy; some into their teens. They have severe physical impairment and sometimes, but not always, severe cognitive impairment, but they are not terminally ill. Most of these children have severe cerebral palsy, the most common cause of permanent disability in children (Meehan et al., 2015, p. 929). The children can experience 'frequent illness due to their increased risk of epilepsy, gastro-intestinal and nutritional problems and respiratory disorders compared with the general childhood population with those children who are most severely motor impaired at the greatest risk' (Meehan et al., 2015, p. 929). They may be dependant in their everyday lives on medical technology, 'with one in ten reliant on a gastronomy feeding tube' (Meehan et al., 2015, p. 929). Despite the complexity of their impairment and health problems, most of the children live at home, attend school and have a wide and varied spectrum of life experiences.

These differences are important ones when best interests decisions are being made. The doctors in my study report much greater uncertainty in prognosis for older children than for infants with degenerative terminal conditions. However, much more is known about the children than the infants. They have a known history, sometimes of more than a decade, not just a medical history, but also a social and educational one. Far more people know them: family, health professionals and professionals.[9] The child's likes and dislikes are known, as are, very likely, how he or she reacts to medical procedures and copes with his or her impairments. Some older and more cognitively able children are able to express an opinion on treatment decisions, including end-of-life decisions. Even younger and less cognitively able children may have communicated preferences through their reactions to past episodes of acute illness and treatment. This seemingly makes the task of exploring the child's best interests 'in the widest sense,'[10] both much easier, as so much more is known, but also perhaps harder precisely because so much more is known, and there is far more to be balanced.

---

[8] The English Court have considered cases concerning the best interests of mostly infants with terminal degenerative conditions, starting with Re B (a minor) (Wardship, Medical Treatment) CA, August 1981, WLR 1421. A good account of the current law can be found in the current RCPCH Guidance; see Larcher (2015).
[9] The voluntary organisation Together For Short Lives lists some of the people likely to be involved in a child's life: http://www.togetherforshortlives.org.uk/assets/0000/1704/Who_s_who.pdf.
[10] *Burke, R (on the application of) vs The General Medical Council*, Rev 1 [2004] EWHC 1879 (Admin) (30 July 2004); per Munby, para. 90.

The doctors

My research involved surveying 32 consultant paediatricians working in tertiary hospitals around the UK, half of them in specialist children's hospitals. All the doctors held senior clinical positions, and some were also clinical managers. Most had significant strategic influence on services regionally and some nationally. A third of the doctors were paediatric intensive care unit (PICU) consultants; just under a third were paediatric neurologists; and the rest were from a range of other paediatric sub-specialities, including neonatology, palliative care, general paediatrics and respiratory medicine. Nine of the doctors also discussed their own and their colleagues' best interests decision-making in extended semi-structured interviews. The surveys and interviews were conducted between 2011 and 2015. The pool of paediatricians was small, but not unusually so for this type of research, (Gallagher, 2006, p. F34). However, it must be noted that as a consequence the results may not be representative of paediatricians across the UK.

The purpose of my research was to discover how paediatricians, by their own accounts, make best interests decisions for disabled children and, in particular, what factors they consider when making those decisions. As a lawyer, I was interested in the role, if any, that the law, rights and ethics play in those decisions. As a parent, I had been intrigued when I had witnessed two consultants examine the same child at the same time, one declaring the child fit and healthy for discharge and the other deciding the child was so critically ill he was in need of immediate intensive care. I wondered how two senior paediatricians could come to such diverse opinions. As a member of numerous national committees drafting guidance relating to the care and death of children and its aftermath for health professionals, I was also interested to learn how doctors used this and other guidance.

Disagreements with other doctors

Perhaps not all together surprisingly, paediatricians, by their own admission, report that best interests decisions for children are some of the most challenging decisions they face.[11] The doctors in my study reported that it is the disagreements as to a child's best interests which make these decisions particularly difficult. However, more doctors reported disagreeing with their medical colleagues than with the child's parents as to a

---

[11] See, for example, Preface by Dr. Hilary Cass, President of RCPCH in Larcher V, 2015.

disabled child's best interests. Seventy-eight per cent (26) of the doctors surveyed reported disagreeing with other doctors, compared with 57.6 per cent (18) of the doctors who reported disagreements with parents. As shall be seen later, these doctors reported responding differently when they disagreed with doctors than with parents.

The doctors answered questions about the factors they consider when making decisions, the weight they attributed to those factors and whom they include in the decision-making process. My sample of 32, in a UK paediatric consultant workforce estimated to have grown between 2013 and 2015 from 3718 to 3996 (RCPCH, 2017, p. 1) is not intended to be generalisable, but rather intended to capture the views of some of the UK's senior consultants making these decisions every day. Their answers perhaps help explain why so many doctors in the study report disagreements with medical colleagues. There was little consensus between doctors as to the factors to be considered, the weight to be put on different factors or whom to include in the decision-making process. For example, some doctors consulted widely, seeking the views of, among others, the child's parents, nurses, teachers and, where possible, the child. Others reported consulting just with medical colleagues or making the decision alone. There was even little consensus as to what doctors meant by terms such as prognosis, quality of life or futility, with the 32 paediatric consultants expressing a range of understandings of these terms. Just as larger studies have found (Cuttini et al., 2000; Richter et al., 2001; Mebane et al., 1999), examination of the doctors' personal and professional characteristics suggested factors such as a doctor's gender, age, religion, sub-specialism, personal experience of disability[12] and duration of practice all potentially influenced how a doctor approached best interests decisions.

Nature of disagreements

The legal judgements[13] in Charlie Gard's case make clear that not only was Charlie different from the children in my study, but so too was the nature of the disagreement. In this case, there was no disagreement among his doctors, which was the most frequent type of disagreement

---

[12] For example, whether the doctor had an impairment him- or herself; or was the parent of a disabled child or had a close disabled relative.
[13] *Great Ormond Street Hospital vs Yates & Gard* [2017] EWHC 972 (Fam); *Yates & Anor vs Great Ormond Street Hospital For Children*, NHS Foundation Trust & Anor (Rev 1) [2017] EWCA Civ 410 (23 May 2017) Gard (A Child), Re [2017] EWHC 1909 (Fam) (24 July 2017); *Gard and Others vs the United Kingdom* – 39793/17 (Decision [2017] ECHR 605 (27 June 2017).

reported by doctors in my study. The first judgement in Charlie's case[14] also makes clear that there was no disagreement among any of the parties that Charlie's quality of life was unsustainable. The disagreement in Charlie's case was whether his quality of life could be improved, not whether it should be sustained.[15] In contrast, in the cases doctors discussed with me, the disagreements were whether it was in a child's best interests to sustain his or her *current* quality of life. Although the disagreement in Charlie's case can be said to be one of quantitative futility, whether a treatment will work; a much more common disagreement for disabled child patients, according to the doctors in my study, is one of qualitative futility, namely, whether given a child's quality of life, it is in his or her best interests to, for example, have antibiotics or be admitted to PICU. It is these qualitative futility decisions that doctors report most commonly cause disagreements.

Disagreements as to qualitative futility are arguably more ethically challenging than arguments of quantitative futility, not least because they are essentially value judgements. It is also unclear who should decide what quality of life is one that should be sustained, meaning that decisions based on these assessments can become life limiting. Medical ethics has grappled with this question for almost four decades. Kennedy (2001) highlighted it, questioning the legitimacy of some doctors' decisions. In relation to end-of-life decisions for infants, he said:

> It is a decision of great moral weight which cannot and should not be left to the discretion of the particular doctor or teams of doctors. There is nothing in the training of a doctor which makes him specially or uniquely competent to make such a decision. (Kennedy, 2001, p. 25)

Current ethical guidance on end-of-life best interests decisions provided to doctors by both the General Medical Council (GMC), the body that registers and regulates all UK doctors, and the Royal College of Paediatrics and Child Health (RCPCH), the body responsible for the development and training of paediatricians in the UK, recognises the subjective nature of qualitative best interests decisions. The RCPCH guidance guides doctors that

> Courts have recognised that quality of life determinations should be based on the individual circumstances of the person, taking account of his or her perceptions without discrimination; quality of life that could be considered intolerable to one who is able-bodied may not be intolerable to one who is born with disability or has developed long-term disability. (Larcher et al., 2015, para 2.3.6)

---

[14] *Great Ormond Street Hospital vs Yates & Gard* [2017] EWHC 972 (Fam); para 48.
[15] *Great Ormond Street Hospital vs Yates & Gard* [2017] EWHC 972 (Fam); para 48.

It acknowledges that 'all decisions about best interests of a child involve value judgements' (Larcher et al., 2015, para. 2.4.2) and recognises that parties involved in a decision may disagree 'because they have different values' (Larcher et al., 2015, para 2.4.2). Guidance from the GMC also cautions doctors: 'You must be careful not to make judgements based on poorly informed or unfounded assumptions about the impact of a disability on a child or young person's quality of life' (General Medical Council, 2013d, p. 96).

Two camps

The doctors in my study suggest that doctors not only bring different values to their best interests decisions but also take very individual approaches to the decisions generally. Each doctor seems to decide him- or herself which factors are relevant, the weight to put on those factors and whom to include in the decision-making process. Indeed, one of the doctors went as far as to say, 'If you have got a dozen respiratory consultants looking at the same child, it is very likely that they would all come to 12 different conclusions'. However, although doctors' decision-making seems to be very individual to a doctor, the doctors in this study did seem to fall into two clear camps. In one camp were doctors, most often but not always those who had long-term relationships with the child and family, who seemed to tailor their decisions to the individual child. In the other camp were doctors who tended to be, but again were not always, acute specialists, called in during a crisis, who did not have long-term relationships with children or families. In their answers, these doctors, perhaps because they did not know the children as individuals, relied much more on set rules or criteria devised by the doctor. For example, one doctor suggested he would not give an intensive care bed to any disabled child who could not perform a particular physical movement. Several doctors suggested that they would withhold certain treatments from children with cognitive impairment.

The disagreements between the doctors seemed to largely be between doctors from these two camps. The first camp criticised the second for making what the first camp described as prejudicial assumptions about a child rather than checking the facts for an individual child. Doctors gave examples of colleagues assuming that a disabled child must have a poor quality of life. In the words of one doctor, 'There is sometimes certainly a sense that you have to go and advocate for your children under your care. PICU staff would otherwise be offering less.' Another doctor described challenging an acute care colleague who decided a disabled child could not have an intensive care bed because he assumed the child was too impaired to attend school, when the child did in fact attend school.

Several doctors voiced fears that some colleagues viewed all disabled children as being the same, making blanket decisions to treat all severely disabled children in a particular way, rather than considering the best interests of individual children on a case-by-case basis, as the law requires (Larcher et al., 2015, para 2.3.6). In the words of one doctor, voicing a concern expressed by several in the study, 'When faced with a child with a lot of special needs ... there is a tendency, you know, [to say,] "oh well they are going to die anyway."' Several doctors in the first camp were particularly critical of their PICU colleagues, although there were also some PICU doctors who expressed similar criticisms of other PICU consultants. One doctor summed up a concern expressed by several:

> I think there is misunderstanding with those in intensive care, that they are supposed to be gatekeepers for the state, to an extent. That is, in my view, absolutely ethically unjustifiable ...
>
> I'm concerned about the idea of treating people according to their type. The idea that there is just a certain type of person who shouldn't be ventilated is meaningless.

The first camp of doctors tended to talk about the positive aspects of a child's life, such as close loving relationships with parents and siblings, whereas the second camp of doctors tended, in contrast, to talk about the burdens of treatment to a child, for example the discomfort of being suctioned or the pain of blood tests. These doctors also stressed the risks of treatment, such as the possibility that a child may become ventilator dependent if ventilated during an acute illness – and indeed the burdens to the child of any physical or cognitive impairments. In essence, the two camps seemed to approach the decision from two sides of a best interests balance sheet,[16] with one looking largely to the benefits of treatments and the other largely to the burdens. Depending on how doctors deal with these disagreements, this could have a positive impact on decision-making, ensuring a wider and fuller examination of a child's best interests, from the different perspectives.

A second distinction to emerge was between older, more experienced, doctors and younger, newly qualified consultants in this study. The older doctors seemed to take a more paternalistic approach, being more inclined to say they made decisions alone or just with other doctors. In contrast, the younger doctors reported consulting widely, seeking the views of nurses, the child's parents and even, in some cases, the child's

---

[16] The English Court has suggested that doctors draw up a best interests balance sheet in which they list the pros and cons of treatment. In *A NHS trust vs MB* [2006] EWHC 507 (Fam) Holman made the balance sheet available in his judgement.

teacher and, where possible, the child. The two generations also expressed different attitudes towards disability discrimination, with several of the older doctors criticising their younger colleagues in this regard. One older doctor voiced her concern that disability discrimination training had led to a change in culture, where younger doctors, she believed, paid too much attention to equality legislation and were too willing to treat disabled children. Another of the older doctors suggested disability training made doctors less questioning and more likely to agree with parents, which he saw as a negative change. In addition, the older doctors tended to suggest that equality legislation encouraged decisions which were not in a child's best interests.

How doctors deal with disagreements with other doctors

As well as describing the disagreements they experienced, the doctors in this study also discussed how they dealt with these disagreements. Some spoke of challenging what they saw as outdated and prejudicial attitudes and correcting misinformation, but these doctors tended to be in the minority. The doctors more commonly spoke of privately disagreeing, but not speaking up to challenging colleagues. They spoke of being respectful of colleagues' different opinions, speaking of a deeply ingrained culture of respecting the autonomy of colleagues' decisions. They expressed a reluctance to challenge opinions, even when they believed them to be fundamentally wrong and would lead to care being withheld or withdrawn from a child. Doctors talked of 'not wanting to rock the boat'. The observations of these doctors suggest a hierarchy of paediatricians, with PICU consultants, seen by many as beyond challenge at the top. Some of the doctors expressed real moral anxiety at not having voiced their opinions; for example, one doctor spoke of sleepless nights thinking of disabled children he believed had died because he had not challenged what he saw as colleagues' prejudicial attitudes towards those children.

Ethical implications

The doctor's challenge here gets to the heart of medical ethics as the 'application of ethical reasoning to medical decision-making' (Herring, 2014, p. 11). Doctors who reported having grave concerns about their colleagues' assessments of a disabled child's best interests seem faced with the choice between two professional ethical obligations: on the one hand, a duty to respect their colleagues' autonomy of clinical judgement; and on the other, a duty to act in a child's best interests. The doctors in my study suggest that (i) this is not an unusual dilemma for a doctor when the best interests of a disabled child are being evaluated, and (ii) it is more common when faced with this dilemma for a doctor to prioritise a colleague's autonomy of clinical judgement over a joint assessment of a disabled child's best interests. However, the doctor's description of sleepless nights, and indeed the way several of the doctors talked about the issue, suggested that not having challenged colleagues has left them with considerable moral anxiety. There will certainly be circumstances where different doctors legitimately come to a different view of a child's best interests because he or she 'may emphasize different principles or assign different weight to principles even when they agree on which principles are relevant' (Beauchamp and Childress, 2009, p. 25). There will also be situations where doctors come to different, but equally ethically sound conclusions, as one will have access to information another does not (Beauchamp and Childress, 2009, p. 25). It also possible to imagine situations where information about a child will simply not be known, as is often the case for infants. However, the situations these doctors described seem slightly but significantly ethically different. They suggest that they are choosing to withhold information from colleagues for fear of 'rocking the boat'. It does seem that there should be an ethical imperative to bring all the information known about a child into a best interests discussion, especially as we have seen the best interests of the child should be the primary concern or paramount.[17] Most particularly, this seems important if doctors believe their colleagues are making wrong or prejudicial assumptions about a child. It seems that moral courage is needed to present the information to their colleagues, who it seems may simply be unaware of it. The same decision may still be made, or the new information could lead to a different decision. At the very least, an ethically sound decision based on all available information and an exploration of the child's best interests in the widest possible terms will have been assured. When the decisions in question concern the life or death of a child, this seems particularly important.

Although, as we have seen, current professional ethical guidance does address best interests decision-making for children, it seems to assume that all doctors with information will add it to the discussion, not withhold it 'for fear of rocking the boat'. The GMC's guidance mentioned

---

[17] Article 3, Paragraph 1, Convention of the Rights of the Child, adopted and opened for signature, ratification and accession by United Nations General Assembly resolution 44/25 of 20 November 1989. Entry into force 2 September 1990, in accordance with article 49, ratified by United Kingdom on 16 December 1991 and came into force on 15 January 1992; see also s. 1 (1) Children Act 1989 (c.41); s.16 (1) Children (Scotland) Act 1995.

earlier 'Good Medical Practice' (General Medical Council, 2013) sets out the legal and ethical duties that doctors owe to their patients. It includes specific 0–18 guidance (General Medical Council, 2013) that guides a doctor caring for a child patient, including as to how best interests decisions should be made. This expressly states that doctors must always act in a child patient's best interests. All doctors are guided to consult widely, including the child's parents (General Medical Council, 2013, p. 8), others close to the child, other health professionals and, where possible, the child (General Medical Council, 2013, pp. 12–13). The guidance tells doctors to 'include what is clinically indicated in a particular case' (General Medical Council, 2013, p. 12), which has the potential to confuse doctors into thinking only clinical issues are relevant. The guidance suggests that where needed legal advice should be sought in individual cases (General Medical Council, 2013, p. 10). The explanatory guidance to GMC 2013 advises further on making 'sound clinical judgements' and doctors are advised that, where 'there are serious differences of opinion between you and the patient, within the healthcare team, or between the team and those close to the patient who lack capacity, about the preferred option for a patient's treatment and care', doctors 'should seek advice or a second opinion from a colleague with relevant experience' (General Medical Council, 2013g, p. 27). As doctors in my study suggest they are reluctant to challenge colleagues, it seems unlikely they would turn to the law in cases of disagreement; indeed, it could well be detrimental to future working relationships.

What is also unclear is the extent to which the doctors making the decisions are even aware of their colleagues' concerns. Most of the doctors in this study suggested that they kept their concerns to themselves. However, just as doctors now have a duty of candour to tell patients and families when they have made an error (General Medical Council, 2013, pp. 8–9), perhaps what is needed is an ethical duty included in GMC guidance requiring doctors to share with colleagues information they believe is important to best interests decisions. Such a duty would perhaps empower reluctant doctors to put forward relevant information and voice concerns. It would arguably help ensure best interests decisions are ethical and indeed legally sound and considered the child's interest in the widest possible way. The current RCPCH guidance, incidentally published after doctors took part in my study, makes it clear that doctors have an individual and collective responsibility to act in a child's best interests (Larcher et al., 2015, para 3.2.1). It also states that 'all members of the treating team need to be part of the decision-making process: their individual views should be sought and accorded due weight' (Larcher et al., 2015, para 3.3.1). The doctors in my study suggest that at least at the time this guidance was published (which updates but retains the same basic principles of earlier guidance published in RCPCH [2004]), this was often not happening. It seems unlikely, particularly as only 17, or 55 per cent, of the doctors in my study reported using guidance when making best interests decisions, and those that did suggested that they do so to justify their actions to others, not to guide them how to make a decision, that doctors' best interests decision-making has greatly changed since.

Disagreements with parents

The doctors in my study also talked about disagreements with parents as to a child's best interests. As reported earlier, fewer doctors (18, or 57.6%) reported disagreeing with parents than with other doctors (26, or 78%). The doctors also said less about the reasons for their disagreements with parents, but several doctors said they thought parents' religious beliefs were a cause of disagreements. Doctors in the second camp were also critical of parents for what they perceived to be parents' unrealistic expectations of medical treatment for their children. Doctors in my study covered a full spectrum of viewpoints as to the role parents should play in end-of-life decisions; from those who saw the decision as solely a decision for doctors, to those who saw it as the parents' decision supported by doctors. Current RCPCH ethical guidance tells doctors that there is a presumption that parents should always be involved in decisions to limit treatment and that parents should always be invited to take part (Larcher et al., 2015, para 2.4.3). However, even when parents are included in the decision-making process, the doctors' accounts suggested that they see the purpose of discussions as being to convince parents to accept the doctors' view of the child's best interests rather than an exchange of viewpoints and information.

Parents' perspective

Although my study did not seek the views of parents, wider research also suggests that parents of disabled children commonly feel pressured by doctors to agree with the doctor's viewpoint as to their child's best interests (Zaal-Schuller et al., 2016, p. 290; Brotherton and Abbott, 2012, p. 590; de Vos, 2015a, p. 197; and Guon, 2014, p. 312). Smith et al.'s (2013) review of 34 studies of the experiences of parents of children with long-term conditions, including 10 studies from the UK, also found that parents reported 'information given quickly with little opportunity for discussion'. Smith et al. (2013, p. 456) along with other studies[18] also reported that 'parents describe difficulties in obtaining information' to enable them to make an informed decision. This does seem to suggest that doctors' perceptions of decision-making discussions with parents, and the extent to which parents feel empowered to express their views in such discussions, may be somewhat different from parents' perceptions.

Doctors' reactions to parents

The two camps of doctors identified here also tended to exhibit different reactions to parents. The first camp tended to talk about parents compassionately, referring to the pain parents suffer seeing their child seriously ill and possibly dying. They tended to speak of the role parents play in supporting and caring for their children and parents' expertise in their child's health. In contrast, the second camp of doctors tended to use very different language, often making moral judgements about parents, for example describing them as 'cruel' or 'selfish' if the 'parents' view as to their child's best interests differed from the doctors'. One doctor, whose comments generally put him in the second camp, described a parent as being 'pathologically ill' when he and the parent disagreed. Indeed, doctors in the second camp were more likely to report disagreements with parents than doctors from the first camp. Although 80 per cent of the PICU consultants in this study who mostly, but not exclusively, fell within the second camp reported disagreements with parents, only 33 per cent of neurologists who mostly, but not exclusively, fell within the first camp tended to do so.

This also echoes the findings of wider studies, which have also found that doctors with long-term relationships with a child and family are less likely to have disagreements with parents at the end of a child's life (Zaal-Schuller et al., 2016, p. 287). Part of the reason for this may be that the doctors who work with the families long term seem to have more of a shared perception of a child with the child's parents than with some of their acute colleagues. Indeed, there are certainly echoes between the concerns doctors in the first camp voiced about the attitudes and opinions of some of their colleagues as to the quality of life of severely disabled children, with the concerns voiced by parents about the perceived negative attitudes of some doctors in other studies. Parental concerns that the lives of disabled children, particularly those with cognitive impairment, are not understood or valued by doctors making end-of-life decisions about

---

[18] See, for example, (Allen KA, 2014).

their child, were widely reported in research studies (Zaal-Schuller et al., 2016, p. 291).

Comments from several of the doctors suggested that rather than using 'best interests' to open up discussions and consider the child's welfare widely, as required by the law and professional ethical guidance, doctors seem to use the term to close down discussions, asserting their clinical expertise and dismissing parents' views as not in the child's best interests, without full discussion. This finding is also echoed in studies of parents' and, more widely, patients' reported experiences of shared decision-making. For example Joseph-Williams et al. (2014) in their systematic review of barriers to shared decision-making found that 'authoritarian or dismissive clinicians who dominate decision-making encounters, do not listen to or respect patient's concerns, or use negative verbal or non-verbal behaviours as a barrier to shared decision-making for many patients' (Joseph-Williams et al., 2014, p. 305).

Doctors' fears

In this study, some of the doctors in the second camp also expressed anxiety and fear that disagreements with parents would lead to the doctor losing his or her GMC registration. One doctor exemplified this by talking of pressure from society forcing doctors to 'overtreat' disabled children against their better judgement. She spoke of feeling pressured to act against a child's best interests to avoid being struck off the GMC register.

Ethical implications of disagreements with parents

These disagreements with parents raise ethical questions in respect of each of the parties. For the child, the same point can be made as was made earlier, to question how ethically sound a decision can be deemed to be if information, in this case known to a parent and pertinent to the decision, is not considered by the decision maker. Turning to the position of the parent, the doctors in my study seemed unclear as to the extent of any ethical duty they had towards a child's parents. RCPCH (2015) makes clear that doctors do have a duty to a child's parents, but is less clear as to the nature and extent of that duty: 'Children's healthcare professionals have an additional duty to the child's family. Part of good paediatric care involves an assessment of the harms and benefits for parents for families as a whole. Challenge may arise when the duty to benefit the child conflicts with a duty to the parents' (Larcher et al., 2015, para 2.4.1). Allen (2014) who studies parents' involvement in decision-making for 'medically complex infants and children', a demographic the children in my study would come within, found that conflict between health professionals and parents 'may negatively affect long-term outcomes both of physical and psychological health of the parents ... Life versus death decision-making can increase parent mortality, mental illness and morbidity' (Allen, 2014, p. 1291).

Some doctors from the first camp in my study suggested that the decision-making process, as much as the final outcome, impacts parents' well-being. The doctors suggested that parents want to be fully involved in the decision to ensure all relevant aspects of the child's life are fully examined and all options are fully explored. Indeed, the few doctors who had been involved in cases which had been referred to court reported that although both families and doctors felt initial concerns at lawyers being involved, they ultimately found the experience helpful and were relieved that the child's best interests had been fully explored and scrutinised. Just as there seems to be a moral imperative to ensure all known information about a child is considered in best interests decisions, so too my own and wider research seem to suggest that it is important for doctors to ensure that parents are fully involved in the decisions. This is important not just to ensure an ethically sound and informed decision is made about the child but also to help safeguard the parents' mental and physical well-being, arguably also an ethically important consideration for doctors involved. Although this chapter has not looked into the issue, it seems likely that a decision-making process fraught with conflict, or where some doctors feel excluded from the decision for whatever reason, is also likely to have detrimental impact on the doctors involved. Indeed, the comment by the doctor about sleepless nights, and the moral anxiety caused to the doctor mentioned earlier, suggests this is the case.

The fear of litigation and of losing their livelihood also seems to cause moral anxiety to a number of the doctors in the second camp. While the anxiety doctors' feel is clearly real, the extent to which this anxiety is well founded does perhaps need further examination. The doctors expressed anxiety at the prospect of losing their registration if they act in what they believed to be the child's best interests rather than doing what parents wished. The GMC statutory purpose is 'to protect, promote and maintain the health and safety of the public by ensuring proper standards in the practice of medicine' (General Medical Council, 2014h) and doctors risk sanction if they fail to follow guidance (General Medical Council, 2013). There is however nothing in the GMC guidance to suggest that a doctor would be sanctioned for acting in what he or she believed to be a child's best interests, indeed, that is what doctors are guided to do (General Medical Council, 2013).

Moreover, even if a parent complained, there seems to be little likelihood that the GMC would investigate. The GMC's annual statistics (General Medical Council, 2015i) reports that 80 per cent of complaints about doctors received from members of the public in 2015 were closed with no investigation being conducted. The statistics do not deal expressly with complaints about best interests decision-making, but such a complaint would seem to fall under the heading of 'Clinical competence and communication and respect for patients allegations' (General Medical Council, 2015i, p. 66). Of these complaints, the GMC report for 2015:

> 92% of investigations involving clinical competence from members of the public resulted in no sanction or warning. Moreover, only a very small percentage of clinical competence investigations resulted in a sanction or a warning; 71% from other doctors and employers and 76% from all others resulted in no sanction or warning (General Medical Council, 2015i, p. 70).

The GMC's statistics suggest that the anxiety some of the doctors in my study expressed about being sanctioned if they 'acted in a child's best interests' against parents' wishes is perhaps disproportionate to any real risk, even if parents were to complain. It is unclear whether the doctors' anxiety is based on a misunderstanding of the guidance, a lack of awareness of the risk of a GMC investigation or is a manifestation of doctors' own moral anxiety about best interests decisions for disabled children generally.

Conclusion

The doctors in my study and the wider literature which has explored parents' perceptions of end-of-life best interests decision-making suggest that despite the ethical guidance available to doctors, the best interests of disabled children in the UK may not always be met, as children's best interests are not always explored in the full and expansive way the courts and ethical guidance say they should be. This chapter has tried to identify some of the reasons for this and suggested that an ethical duty on doctors to disclose information they know about a child may be needed. As suggested in Charlie Gard's case,[19] third-party assistance, perhaps in the form of mediation, is needed to ensure that a child's best interests are fully explored without disagreements arising. It seems clear that barriers do exist, many of which seem to be in relation to communication between doctors, and between doctors and parents. These, it seems, are preventing

---

[19] Great Ormond Street Hospital vs Yates & Gard [2017] EWHC 972 (Fam); para 130.

the ethically sound examination of some disabled children's best interests, possibly to their detriment as well as that of their parents and the doctors involved.

References

Allen, K.A. (2014) Parental decision-making for medical complex infants and children. An integrated literature review. *International Journal of Nursing Studies*, 51(9), pp. 1289–1304.

Beauchamp, T.L. and Childress, J.F. (2009) *Principles of Biomedical Ethics*. Oxford: Oxford University Press.

British and Irish Legal Information Institute. http://www.bailii.org/datbases. html (accessed 11 February 2018).

Brotherton, A. and Abbott, J. (2012) Mothers' process of decision making for gastrostomy placement. *Qualitative Health Research*, 22(5), pp. 587–94

Children Act (1989). http://www.legislation.gov.uk/ukpga/1989/41/section/16 (accessed 11 February 2018).

Children (Scotland) Act (1995). https://www.legislation.gov.uk/ukpga/1995/36/ contents (accessed 11 February 2018).

Cuttini, M., Nadai, M., Hansen, G., de Leeuw, R., Lenoir, S., Persson, J., Reba-gliato, M. et al. (2000) End of life decisions in neonatal intensive care: Physicians' self-reported practices in seven European countries. EURONIC Study Group. *Lancet*, 355(9221), pp. 2112–18.

de Vos, M.A., Bos, A.P., Plotz, F.B., van Heerde, M., de Graffe, B.M., Tates, K., Truog, R.D. et al. (2015a) Talking with parents about end-of-life decisions for their children. *Pediatrics*, 135(2), pp. 465–76.

de Vos, M.A., Seeber, A.A., Gevers, S.K., Bos, A.P., Gevers, F. and Willems, D.L. (2015b) Parents who wish no further treatment for their child. *Journal of Medical Ethics*, 41(2), pp. 195–200.

Gallagher, K. (2006) *Teaching Adolescent Writers*. Portland, ME: Stenhouse Publishers.

General Medical Council (2013) Standards and ethics guidance for doctors. https://www.gmc-uk.org/publications/standards_guidance_for_doctors.asp (accessed 11 February 2018).

Guon, J. (2014) Our children are not a diagnosis: the experience of parents who continue their pregnancy after a prenatal diagnosis of trisomy 13 or 18. *American Journal Medical Genetics*, 164A(2), pp. 308–18.

Hansard. (2007). Lord St. John of Fawsley, (2007) *'House of Lords Debate'*, 31 January, Column 236. https://publications.parliament.uk/pa/ld200607/ ldhansrd/text/70131-0002.htm (accessed 11 February 2018).

Herring, J. (2014) *Medical Ethics and Law*. Oxford: Oxford University Press.

Joseph-Williams, N., Elwyn, G. and Edwards, A. (2014) Knowledge is not power for patients: a systematic review and thematic synthesis of patient-reported barriers and facilitators to shared decision making. *Patient Education and Counselling*, 94(3), pp. 291–309.

Kennedy, I. (2001), *Treat Me Right, Essays in Medical Law and Ethics*. Oxford: Oxford University Press.

Larcher, V., Craig, F., Bhogal, K., Wilkinson, D. and Brierley, J. (2015) Making decisions to limit treatment in life-limiting and life-threatening conditions in children: a framework for practice. *Archives of Disease in Childhood*, 100, pp. s1–s23.

Mebane, E.W., Oman, R.F., Kroonen, L.T. and Goldstein, M.K. (1999) The influence of physician race, age, and gender on physician attitudes toward advance care directives and preferences for end-of-life decision-making. *Journal of the American Geriatrics Society*, 47(5), pp. 579–91.

Meehan, E., Freed, G.L., Reid, S.M., Williams, K., Sewell, J.R., Rawicki, B. and Reddihough, D.S. (2015) Tertiary paediatric hospital admissions in children and young people with cerebral palsy. *Child: Care, Health and Development*, 41(6), pp. 928–37.

Royal College of Paediatrics and Child Health (RCPCH). (2004). *Withholding or withdrawing life-sustaining treatment in children—a framework for practice*, 2nd edn. London: RCPCH.

Royal College of Paediatrics and Child Health (RCPCH). (2017) Medical Workforce Census 2015. https://www.rcpch.ac.uk/sites/default/files/user31401/2015%20RCPCH%20Workforce%20Census%20FULL.pdf (accessed 12 February 2018).

Richter, J., Eisemann, M. and Zgonnikova, E. (2001) Doctors' authoritarianism in end-of-life treatment decisions. A comparison between Russia, Sweden and Germany. *Journal of Medical Ethics*, 27(3), pp. 186–91.

Smith, J., Cheater, F. and Bekker, H. (2013) Parents experiences of living with a child with a long-term condition: a rapid structured review of the literature, *Health Expectations*, 18(4), pp. 452–74.

Together for Short Lives (n.d.) Family Resources, Who is Who, Together for Short Lives. http://www.togetherforshortlives.org.uk/assets/0000/4092/Who_s_who.pdf (accessed 11 February 2018).

Zaal-Schuller, I.H., Willems, D.C., Ewals, F.V.P.M., van Goudoever, J.B. and de Vos, M.A. (2016) How parents and physicians experienced end-of-life decision-making for children with profound intellectual & multiple disabilities. *Research in Developmental Disabilities*, 59, pp. 283–93.

8

Decision-making and reciprocity: public and private considerations

Hazel Biggs and Angela Fenwick

Discussion

The preceding three chapters explored the ethical issues raised by women sharing and donating breast milk, prioritising healthcare for armed forces veterans, and best interest decision-making for children. While these are distinct areas, they all raise questions about the boundary between private and public practices and the extent to which an activity can, or should, be considered private. Alongside this, decision-making and reciprocity are prominent themes running throughout the section.

In Chapter 5, Sally Dowling delved into the practice of sharing leftover breast milk, a topic fraught with cultural meanings and ethical concerns centring on quality assurance and safety. She usefully compared women who informally share their breast milk – for example through online networks – with those who donate to more formal regulated networks, for example for premature babies. The latter is often constructed as an altruistic act of saving a life, whereas the former raises concerns about potentially risking the lives of the recipient babies. One tends to be publically regulated – and approved of – whereas the other is informal and essentially a private transaction between women. Dowling explored the extent to which the act of sharing may be seen as a reciprocal arrangement among women: a type of mother-to-mother support – facilitated by the internet – or an 'act of care', which may be regarded as altruistic. Given the evidence to support breast milk over formula milk, she asks whether such currently informal sharing practices ought to be more widely facilitated or regulated through public health bodies.

The issues and questions raised by this piece in many ways go to the core of mothering responsibilities and women's ability to care for their offspring according to their own ethical values. At a time when public health messages promote the undoubted benefits of breastfeeding, and women may feel demonised if they cannot provide breast milk themselves, either for physical or social reasons, it would seem unfortunate if women were condemned for providing or receiving breast milk through these sharing practices. Regulating such practices runs the risk of locating them in the public domain and perhaps introducing regulatory barriers into the process that could be seen as tantamount to interference in women's decisions about the use of their bodies and their bodily products, and may lead to reduced supply. On the other hand, allowing breast milk sharing to remain an essentially private concern, where women assess the possible risks for themselves and balance the competing harms and benefits for their children, as they do in most other parenting decisions, could be anathema to the state-implemented public health agenda.

Hilary Engward, in Chapter 6, introduced us to the UK Armed Forces Covenant (2011), a statutory regime which gives armed forces veterans (defined, it seems, as anyone who has served a minimum of one day in uniform) the entitlement to receive priority healthcare within the National Health Service (NHS) for injuries relating to their service. The Covenant seems to be underpinned by the notion that veterans should be compensated for sacrifices made as part of their military service that have disadvantaged them when compared to other citizens: essentially, a reciprocal relationship between the state – on behalf of the public, whom the veteran serves – and the individual veteran. The recognition of this sacrifice by the government may be reflective of the fact that veterans sign up to a loss of liberty, subsumed to the collective, and that they are also subject to harms resulting from wars carried out in the state's name. We might speculate that the fact introduction of the Covenant was at a time when service men and women have experienced combat situations, such as in Iraq and Afghanistan, which were not necessarily envisaged when signing up, was influential in its inception. But is this potential inequity in access to healthcare justifiable?

Engward explores the arguments against such a system of prioritisation in healthcare, for example that others, such as firefighters, can also come to harm in their pursuit of saving lives, but concludes that the difference between firefighters and veterans is the level of sacrifice made by veterans is much greater and also unique in our society, which gives rise to an ethical justification for priority access to healthcare. However, she includes the caveat that it is only so if the injury comes from service '*and* only when no other patient with more urgent medical needs requires attention'. Essentially, this conclusion holds that if all else is equal, then the veteran should be given priority. This, in reality, might mean that veterans are only rarely given priority, as decisions about who should be treated first are judgements about clinical need: it seems unlikely that two or more people would present with exactly the same clinical need at the same time. To what extent, then, is the covenant illusionary, fulfilling a political agenda rather than offering a genuine benefit to the veteran community? If the promised benefits do not materialise, the ethical concern shifts from one of reciprocity, leading to possible unequal access to healthcare in the general population, to one of false hope and thwarted expectations in the veteran community.

In the final chapter of this section, Zoe Picton-Howell turned attention to the decision-making process in relation to the best interests of children, and specifically to the implications of disagreements about what might be in an individual child's best interests. Her piece is timely because during writing the Charlie Gard case at Great Ormond Street Hospital hit the headlines; although her focus was on older children with a disability or chronic condition, some of the issues raised are still pertinent. Picton-Howell conducted surveys and interviewed a small number of paediatricians about their approach to the decision-making process. She found that disagreements between clinicians often arose from individuals' differing value systems and the weighting they gave to the different criteria used for best interests assessments. Furthermore, they dealt with these in different ways: some not wishing to express their viewpoint publicly – because of hierarchy or fear of challenging colleagues' opinions – what they privately had concluded, which sometimes led to moral distress. Other types of disagreement were between doctors and parents as to what was in their child's best interests. In such circumstances, she found that some clinicians thought their role was to persuade parents to their position. She concludes that the best interests of the children with disabilities could be more thoroughly thought through and argues for the use of third-party mediation when disagreements do arise.

Best interests is a complex concept which involves a subjective component, and it is not surprising that clinicians disagree with one another or with parents when making such assessments. When disagreements arise, the law is the final arbiter, and legal precedent makes it clear that best interests reflect a range of factors, including social and welfare considerations as well as clinical aspects, which must be weighed in the balance to determine the *best* course of action. Tensions are therefore almost inevitable as parents and clinicians are likely to prioritise different factors. Picton-Howell, however, raises interesting questions about the extent to which information that surrounds such decisions should be made public. Within a hospital setting, such an approach should involve the multidisciplinary team and include doctors and parents, but may not always be transparent and is necessarily not publically accessible to protect confidentiality. In a court case, a judge will construct a balance sheet in the process of making a best interests assessment, the outcome of which is then recorded in publicly available case reports, for transparency. However, once the judicial process is underway, unlike the parents, who can waive anonymity, the healthcare professionals involved are unable to comment in the public domain, and this public–private divide can potentially lead to very one-sided reporting.

Although the topics of these three chapters appear rather disparate, they do in fact explore similar ethical issues in relation to reciprocity, altruism and the public–private divide. Each raises questions about the role of the individual in society and more particularly in relation to access to aspects of healthcare, such as breast milk, specialist medical treatment or life-prolonging care. As such, the section provides a lens through which to try to better understand how these ethical concerns relate to the provision of healthcare more generally.

PART 3

New Voices

Nursing the Nation[1, 2]

Molly Case

> A woman comes in,
> too young to bear this;
> she's got a disease that will make her miss –
> her daughter's wedding day,
> her first grandchild being born.
> How would that feel, to have that all torn
> away from you?
>
> I can't answer that question,
> it's not my place to say,
> but I can tell you what we did for her,
> how we helped her get through the day.
> A cup of tea there and one for all her family,
> as they came, throughout the night,
> what a sight; there were loads of them.
> To help her fight the awful pain of it,
> paying last visits, we wouldn't let them miss it –
> farewell from a brother,
> last kisses with their mother –
> holiest love, love like no other.

---

[1] This poem was written as reflex, a knee-jerk reaction to a portrayal of our profession in the media that wasn't representative of the majority of us. I wanted to highlight all the small but wonderful things we do as nurses that sometimes go un-noticed, the cups of tea, the hand holds. It is these 'small' things that leave a lasting impression on somebody's life.

[2] Nursing the Nation and Welcome to Paradise © Molly Case 2015, used with permission of Burning Eye Books.

Maybe there's bad ones,
no doubt that there are,
but for this list I'm writing
we don't want the same tar-brush,
crushing our careers before they've even started;
how could you say this
about people so big-hearted?

Who would have thought we'd be having to defend?
We don't do this for our families,
we don't do this for our friends,
but for strangers.
Because this is our vocation
and we're sick and tired
of being told we don't do enough for this nation.
So listen to us, hear us goddamn roar;
you say we're not doing enough?
Then we promise we'll do more.
This time, next time,
there's nothing we can't handle,
even if you bring us down,
show us scandal, scandal, scandal.
You remember that man covered in burns head to toe?
I don't think you do
'cause you were on that TV show:
lipgloss-kissed women on daytime TV,
come into our world, see things that we see.

One lady, passing, had no relatives to stay.
We sang her to sleep, let angels take her away.
Were you there that day when we held her hand?
Told her nothing would harm her,
that there was a higher plan.
Saw her face as she remembered a faith she'd once held,
watched her breath in the room as she finally exhaled.

Why don't you meet us? Come, shake our hands.
Try to fit it in between having tea with your fans.
Your hands are so soft and mine are cracked.
Why don't you let us on air?
Let us air the facts.

We've washed and shrouded people
that we've never known,
pinned flowers to the sheet
and told them they're still not alone.
Shown families to the faith room
and watched them mourn their dead,
then got back to work, bathed patients, made beds.
Hindus, Muslims, Jews and Sikhs,
Buddhists and Christians and just people off the street,
we've cared for them all and we love what we do,
we don't want a medal, we just want to show you.
So listen to us, hear us goddamn roar;
you say we're not doing enough?
Then we promise we'll do more.

9

We need to talk about ethics and social media: a conversation

Rebecca J. Hogue and Marie Ennis-O'Connor

Introduction

As more people share personal illness narratives in online blogs and other social media, the blurring between public and private raises ethical questions. Health researchers are now using this wealth of unsolicited information about patient lived experience as data for their research. Is information shared freely available to researchers simply because it is available on a public website? Should personal information always be treated as confidential even when the person self-discloses on social media? What are the ethics of collecting and analysing peoples' stories or observing peoples' online behaviour without asking for consent to be part of a research study? In an age when technology has outpaced the ethical underpinnings of research and the culture surrounding privacy has changed profoundly, we need to rethink how to do this research in a manner that is ethical and responsive to participants' wishes.

This chapter takes the form of a conversation between the authors on the ethical obligations of researchers using patient-generated social media data in their studies. The authors are both cancer bloggers and active participants in Twitter cancer communities. Further, the international nature of social media–based research is reflected by the authors, as Marie is Irish and Rebecca is a Canadian living in California, United States. Although patients also use forums and groups (e.g. Facebook groups) for social support, this chapter focuses on publicly available blogs and Twitter communities. Although there is guidance provided on the ethical use of forums for research (e.g. Kozinets, 2015), there is a lack of guidance and conflicting opinions on how to use blogs and microblogs such as Twitter in research studies. The conversation begins with a discussion on the ways in which blogs can be used in an ethical manner by researchers, followed by a conversation on the use of Twitter in research. We conclude with practical guidelines on how researchers may ethically use public blogs and Twitter data in research.

What do we mean by ethical use of social media in research?

Rebecca: In an academic sense, ethics is defined as 'the discipline dealing with what is good and bad and with moral duty and obligation' (Oxford, https://www.merriam-webster.com/dictionary/ethic). That being said, in academia we often equate ethics with *procedural ethics*, that is, the process required by the institution to approve the research project. Descriptions of proposed research studies are submitted to an ethics review board for ethical approval. However, I'm concerned that procedural ethics aren't enough, especially when research is about patient experience. What is considered ethical in a clinical setting doesn't necessarily make a lot of sense when conducting research studies on patient experience using social media. When you think about *ethical use*, what does that mean to you, Marie?

Marie: Social media allow for the gathering of a rich source of unsolicited user-generated data that were previously unavailable to researchers, and that's exciting, but this opportunity should be matched by a responsibility to ensure that the ways in which these data are obtained and reused is done in an ethical manner. Because social media are still relatively new and they are dynamic and constantly evolving, at this time there is no clear ethical framework for how to use them in research. Research ethics boards serve an important function, which is to protect research participants. However, most have not kept pace with emerging trends in social media. When it comes to making decisions to approve (or not) this kind of research, ethics boards are either drawing on traditional ethics frameworks (e.g. randomised control trial protocols) or situating social media within a broader framework of internet research (e.g. the Association of Internet Researcher Ethical Framework, https://aoir.org/ethics/). There are nuanced and complex differences, and it's time to recognise that social media bring new contextual challenges to research.

Rebecca: I agree. I've seen first-hand how some ethics boards approve the use of social media as data without a clear understanding of what social media are. Just because the research ethics board determines that a study is exempt from review because the data are publicly available on the internet, does not necessarily mean that the research is exempt from ethical consideration. Research ethics board approval is a minimum bar that does not necessarily deal with the moral implications of research.

How do we use blogs ethically in research?

Rebecca: Before we start, I want to make sure we both have the same understanding of what illness blogs are. I define blogs as self-published, public digital journals. Blogs are used by patients to report on their lived experience with illness. Typically, *illness blogs* contain a chronological series of short stories, known as *blog posts*. Although there is no required format for blog posts, in illness blogs they typically represent a single event, experience or opinion. The collection of blog posts, brought together, form the larger blog. Further, a collection of blogs surrounding a similar topic is known as a *blogosphere*. It is common practice within the blogosphere to refer to subsets of the community based upon the topic of given blogs; for example, education-related blogs are considered part of the *edu-blogosphere*, and a collection of *breast cancer blogs* are referred to as the *breast cancer blogosphere*.[1] Marie, does that align with your understanding of blogs and what made you start blogging?

Marie: Yes, I agree with your definition. I started writing my blog after I had finished treatment for breast cancer. At the time, there was very little written about what happens after treatment ends, and I wanted to share my experience with others. I realised about a year into writing the blog, that my story could provide a unique insight into the long-term impact of cancer. The kind of information about the lived experience of cancer that I, and other bloggers like me, were sharing online couldn't be found anywhere else. These blogs provide an unparalleled opportunity to develop a richer understanding of what it means to be diagnosed with, and live with, cancer. In these blogs, you find descriptions of real-time experiences, and I think that's an incredible gift to researchers and healthcare practitioners. I encouraged nurses, doctors, students and researchers to read my blog and similar others. Becky, you started your blog right after your diagnosis. What inspired you to blog about your breast cancer experience?

Rebecca: I began blogging in the first few days after diagnosis. At that time, it was too hard to say the words. I just couldn't talk about it. I was not ready for telephone conversations, but my family and friends needed to know what was happening. I also had a compulsion to write. I still have that compulsion. It is my therapy. It is how I process my thoughts and ideas. But for me, writing has always needed an audience. I've never been able to write for the sake of writing. I've always needed to write for someone – or write to teach someone.

---

[1] Two examples of breast cancer blogs are http://BCBecky.com and https://journeyingbeyondbreastcancer.com/.

As a researcher and illness blogger, I've read many published research papers that feel like they are taking advantage of the accessibility of blogs and Twitter chats as publicly available resources, but the researchers appear to forget that there are people behind the blogs and tweets (e.g. Bock, 2013; Weber and Solomon, 2008). Marie, what do you think?

Marie: My initial enthusiasm for encouraging the use of blogs in research became tempered with a concern about how this information was actually being used, and how I and other bloggers felt about this. I realised the issue was far more complex than I had first thought and that we all need to take a step back and explore the ethical issues associated with using blogs for research. For instance, I began to have concerns about how we treat the concept of private versus public data. Just because something is publicly available on the internet, is it okay to use such data freely for research purposes? Do we as bloggers have any right to expect any degree of privacy? Illness bloggers frequently write emotive posts, and some patients may be particularly vulnerable, so we should be mindful of this. Privacy is not a simple binary concept; rather, it is more nuanced and complex. What are the issues that concern you, Becky?

Rebecca: Another issue that I see that is related is when quotes are taken out of context. The tradition of research reporting often requires concise language, and it is subject to restrictions on length. Researchers are looking for the perfect quote to fit their argument, and they don't always have space to include the complete context. Direct quotes taken out of context may potentially pose harm to the blogger or tweeter being quoted. Are there other issues that concern you?

Marie: I am concerned with the issue of asking participants for consent. Traditionally, consent is built into research design (e.g. consent forms, boxes to be ticked), but social media–based research often involves collecting and analysing data without consent being sought. An important element of consent in research is ensuring that participants are aware of how their data is being used. As a blogger, do you make any explicit statements about consenting to researchers using your data?

Rebecca: Yes, I give researchers permission but also ask that they tell me about it.[2] Further, Bochner and Riggs (2014) recommend that 'researchers ought to accept an ethical obligation to give something important back

---

[2] For example, 'If you are a researcher, you are welcome to use my blog as data for your research as long as you inform me via email (rhogue@pobox.com) or by leaving a comment on this page. I ask that you attribute quotes directly to me, linking back to my blog, and that you share your research results with me. I reserve the right to ask you to use a different quote. This statement can be used as informed consent.' (http://bcbecky.com/About)

to the people they study and write about' (p. 201). Blog data were created for a purpose, and that purpose was not research, so the creators did not consent for research use (Kozinets, 2015). Blogging takes a lot of work. For many bloggers, it is a labour of love that is completely unpaid and often unrecognised. As researchers who benefit from the freely available data provided in blogs, we should at least acknowledge the contributions bloggers make to our research. Personally, I see no problem with using one, two, even three blog posts without asking consent, but if the researcher is downloading the entire blog for data analysis, then I see that as a 'secondary use of data',[3] and as such, the researcher should use the processes set out by the ethics research board established for secondary use of data.[4]

Another area of concern that I'm seeing is that researchers and ethics boards confuse the research participant with a patient. A research participant in a clinical trial is receiving treatment and is therefore classified as a patient, whereas a research participant in a social media–based study is not receiving treatment from the research organisation and therefore is not a patient in that context. I see this as incorrect context blurring because there is a duty of privacy to patients when giving healthcare, that is not applicable when using public social media data. This incorrect assumption of social media participant as patient happens frequently (e.g. de Boer and Slatman, 2014). This gets even more clouded when research ethics boards declare blog data as public that does not require procedural ethics approval, but then the researchers conceptualise blog data as patient data and seek to anonymise it to protect the identity of patients.

Marie: I know you feel strongly about the practice of anonymising the voices of bloggers. Tell me some more about this.

Rebecca: I see this as issue with attribution, particularly around the experiences of bloggers, as they intentionally want their voices heard, and in some cases researchers try to anonymise direct quotes (e.g. Keim-Malpass et al., 2013). Direct quotes of internet data cannot be truly anonymised meaning that any direct quotes can be entered into an internet search tool and the original source can be found (Kozinets, 2015).

---

[3] The concept of 'secondary use of data' relates to data that are collected or created for a purpose that is different from research. The rules associated with secondary use of data differ across nations, disciplines and organisations.

[4] For example, the NHS Health Research Authority explicitly exempts from review research that is 'Research limited to secondary use of information previously collected in the course of normal care (without an intention to use it for research at the time of collection), provided that the patients or service users are not identifiable to the research team in carrying out the research' (NHS n.d.), however social media data is identifiable and therefore would not be automatically exempt.

But I also am challenged by this practice as a blogger. If I publish in a newspaper article or book, then proper attribution occurs. I think of the publishing of a blog post as parallel to this. I strongly believe that proper attribution of blogs is appropriate. However, I see guidance such as that provided by Denecke et al. (2015), who state that 'preserving patient anonymity when citing Internet content is crucial for research studies' (p. 137). This interpretation of the contributor to social media as patient demonstrates how health researchers sometimes confuse the research participant for a patient.

There are different privacy rights and concerns between research participants and patients. In research, the participant has a right to be identified if he or she chooses to be. Bloggers are choosing to make their words public, and treating them like anonymous patients is misguided. I have observed cases where researchers anonymise blog quotes from bloggers who have since died. I find this especially problematic, as the researchers are not honouring the words of a dead person's legacy. In my opinion, blogs should be appropriately attributed. I think of it as honouring the voices of those who have chosen to share their experiences publicly.

Marie: If I understand you right, it is a question of who gets to choose what happens with the blog data. Is it an ethics board, the researcher or the blogger? I believe it is an ethical imperative for a researcher to ask the owner of the blog how he or she wants to be identified in research.

How do we use Twitter ethically in research?

Rebecca: Let's move on to Twitter now. How would you explain what Twitter is to someone who is not familiar with it?

Marie: Twitter is a micro-blogging platform where users post and interact with messages known as 'tweets,' which are restricted to 280 characters. Registered users can post tweets and interact with other users, but those who are unregistered can only read them. Tweets are publicly visible by default, but senders can choose to keep tweets visible to just their followers. Users can group tweets together by topic by using hashtags (words or phrases prefixed with a '#' sign). A Twitter chat is a public Twitter conversation around one unique hashtag. This hashtag allows you to follow the discussion and participate in it. Twitter chats are usually recurring and based on specific topics to regularly connect people with these interests. You'll find Twitter chats in most disease areas, for example #BCSM, which stands for breast cancer social media.

Rebecca: You blog and use Twitter; do you use them in different ways?

Marie: While I use my blog to delve deeper into my lived experience of breast cancer, Twitter is where I turn to when I am looking for answers to my questions and want to connect in real-time to others. I see it as my personal learning network, and one of the things I love most about it is how individuals can come together in a Twitter conversation – not just patients, but the wider healthcare community. We are both active in Twitter conversations related to our experiences of breast cancer. Do you think there is a difference in how Twitter and blog data should be treated in research?

Rebecca: Context becomes an important issue when using data from Twitter. While the 280 character limit makes the conversation more concise, it also makes it easy for researchers and community participants to take things out of context. Often in Twitter communities you need to follow a conversation over several tweets to appreciate the context of the conversation. Care needs to be taken to ensure that the researcher is not de-contextualising the tweets, which could potentially cause damage to the person who tweeted. Strictly speaking, Twitter data are public; however, members of specific communities will not know that their tweets may be used for research purposes. This brings us back to the idea of informed consent.

Marie: For me, informed consent is a key ethical issue in conducting research using Twitter conversations as data. Informed consent means that a person knowingly and in a clear way gives consent (Armiger, 1997).

Rebecca: What can researchers do to get consent from Twitter communities?

Marie: It's about being transparent and up front from the start. Every Twitter chat has a founder or moderator – someone who identifies him- or herself at the start of each chat – so I recommend researchers contact this person to discuss how they could work with the moderator to further their research. One suggestion I have is for the researcher to become a guest moderator, and the focus of the chat to be the topic of their research. The researcher can then ask questions of participants during the chat, making it clear from the outset that this may be used as research data and explaining the consent procedure. This gives individuals an opportunity to opt out of the chat or ask that their tweets are not used. What do you think about the need for permission to use specific tweets in research reports?

Rebecca: Personally, I always ask the person who tweeted if I can use his or her specific tweet in my research report. It is easy to send a tweet to an individual and ask for permission to use that particular tweet.

Marie: But is this absolutely necessary?

Rebecca: No, it is not necessary; rather, I think it is an important courtesy. If someone is using a specific tweet of mine within his or her conference presentation, I would like to know. I might also be going to that conference, so it may impact me if the tweet is used. Contacting the tweeter also helps me as a researcher, as it connects me to work that others are doing in the same field. I've observed the practice of taking the tweet and blurring out the name of the person who posted it and those who retweeted it. Similar to direct quoting blog resources, you cannot anonymise direct quotes of tweets.

Conclusion

Rather than prescribing a set of approved practices, we offer the following set of questions to prompt reflection about ethical decision-making when using blogs and tweets:

> Considering the paradox between public and private in social media, do we need a new definition of what informed consent means?

> Given the public nature of blogs and tweets, do bloggers and tweeters have a right to privacy?

> What are the potential consequences of stripping data of personally identifiable information?

> How do we ensure that social media data are kept in context when used for research?

> If an ethics board deems no formal consent is required, should the researcher still seek the participants' consent?

> Who benefits from the study – do the participants? If not, what greater benefit justifies the potential risks?

In answering these questions, there isn't a one-size-fits-all recommendation; rather, ethical decision-making is best approached contextually. Following on from our earlier conversation, here is a summary of our key considerations:

> Ethical approaches to publicly available information must include a consideration of the contextual nature of sharing and users' understandings of privacy.

➤ When using blogs as data, refer to the blog's 'About' page to see if there is an explicit consent statement.

➤ Sending an email and commenting directly on the blog are usually effective ways to ask permission.

➤ If the blogger has died, ensure you are correctly quoting and attributing the work, so as not to be taking away the blogger's voice. Note that if a loved one is maintaining the blog, it is appropriate to ask the loved one for permission to use the blog content.

➤ It is fine to use quotes from one or two blog posts, but if you are using an entire blog as a data source, that constitutes secondary use of data and should follow the appropriate protocols for secondary use of data.

➤ Before using Twitter community data, ask the moderator of the community for permission. You can tweet to the community to determine who needs to be asked or informed.

➤ As tweets can easily be taken out of context, before using a specific tweet in a conference presentation or research report, reach out to the tweeter to ask permission.

In conclusion, we hope this chapter proves helpful to researchers concerned with the ethical challenges of using social media data in research. Because social media is constantly evolving, ethical guidelines have to be regularly reviewed. Above all, remember that behind every blog and tweet is a real person.

References

Armiger, B. (1997) No ethics in nursing research: profile, principles perspective. *Nursing Research*, 26(5), pp. 330–33.

Bochner, A. and Riggs, N.A. (2014) *Practicing Narrative Inquiry*. http://www.oxfordhandbooks.com/view/10.1093/oxfordhb/9780199811755.001.0001/oxfordhb-9780199811755.

Bock, S. (2013) Staying positive: women's illness narratives and the stigmatized vernacular. *Health, Culture and Society*, 5(1). http://hcs.pitt.edu/ojs/index.php/hcs/article/view/125.

de Boer, M. and Slatman, J. (2014) Blogging and breast cancer: narrating one's life, body and self on the Internet. *Women's Studies International Forum*, 44, pp. 17–25.

Denecke, K., Bamidis, P., Bond, C., Gabarron, E., Househ, M., Lau, A.Y.S., Mayer, M.A. et al. (2015) Ethical issues of social media usage in healthcare. *IMIA Yearbook*, 10(1), pp. 137–47.

Keim-Malpass, J. et al. (2013) Young women's experiences with complementary therapies during cancer described through illness blogs. *Western Journal of Nursing Research*, 35(10), pp. 1309–24. http://journals.sagepub.com/doi/10.1177/0193945913492897.

Kozinets, R.V. (2015) *Netnography: Redefined*, 2nd edn. Los Angeles, CA: Sage Publications.

NHS Health Research Authority (NHSHRA), Governance arrangements for research ethics committees. https://www.hra.nhs.uk/planning-and-improving-research/policies-standards-legislation/governance-arrangement-research-ethics-committees/ (accessed 26 June 2018).

Weber, K.M. and Solomon, D.H. (2008) Locating relationship and communication issues among stressors associated with breast cancer. *Health Communication*, 23 (March 2015), pp. 548–59.

10

Patients as leaders: reflections on identity, equality and power

Dominic Stenning, with Julie Wintrup

Introduction

This chapter draws on Dominic's experience of working in co-production of healthcare, in which patients and service users work alongside others to design, implement and evaluate services. Collaborating with professional and strategic decision makers, seeing projects come to fruition, and influencing patient care in direct ways, are discussed by Dominic and Julie using an interview style.[1] The benefits of co-production work are discussed along with the personal costs and risks. The effects of working with others to improve services are reflected upon in terms of consolidating a sense of identity as a worker and contributor, and of developing knowledge and insight into issues of equality and the sharing of power. Good practice that is inclusive and fair, and understands the complex and contingent nature of co-production, is discussed.

How did you become involved in co-production of health services, Dominic?

I had many good, bad and – mainly – mediocre experiences of health services, and wanted to change the system I had grown up accessing on and off all my life. I experienced mental illness from childhood and subsequently drug addiction. After my father, who was a general practitioner, died of pancreatic cancer in 1998, my heroin use spiralled out of control,

---

[1] Dominic also blogs at https://patientleader.wordpress.com/about/, and his Twitter username is @PatientLeader.

but after 10 years of heavy drug use, I started a long road to recovery. After getting clean in 2007, I've since been rebuilding my life. But like a lot of people with a mental health condition, I also have physical health problems. I have curvature of the spine, a condition I've had since birth. Two years after getting clean, I was the innocent victim of a car crash in December 2008. My injuries included damage to the part of my back that worked – the lumbar spine – so standing or sitting for periods of time is extremely painful, and my mobility is limited.

After a few bleak years, I started to recover again and got involved with my local NHS trust. In 2013, I helped form The Recovery College East with Cambridgeshire and Peterborough NHS Foundation Trust, which embedded a strong focus on co-production (see *Road to Recovery: Our Stories of Hope* by Gilfoyle and Hodge). I found that working with professionals, policy makers and managers to improve health services could be very rewarding. You realise you have insider knowledge of healthcare, but more importantly, you bring a unique, personal life experience that's meaningful and mostly valued by others, and includes coping and managing with multiple health problems. Being a member of a family that supports one another through difficult times, learning practical tasks such as managing medication and how to get the right type of help in particular circumstances, thinking about how best to organise our lives and our responsibilities, thinking about the future and preserving our lives together no matter what – these are the important things in my life and are all relevant to co-production. They can't be put in a box and called 'my story', told in the past tense. I'm in the middle of it – it's my life, not a 'walk-on part' in someone else's presentation or event.

So working with the Recovery College made me realise I had important, deep knowledge of how to manage pain while recovering from addiction and working out medication regimes, differentiating between symptoms and learning what was most helpful to staying well. At the same time, I started to understand that this kind of knowledge isn't respected or given status. I started to read research articles and policy guidance, and asked myself how I could use my experiential, insider knowledge to the benefit of others. I knew I could identify and empathise with others trying to do the same thing, and often thought about those struggling to recover without family or medical support, like me throughout my life, as I know how tough it is when you fall through the cracks and the system lets you down. I could see that services and individual professionals were often trying hard and doing some things really well, but I knew too that gaps, brick walls and poor practices were all too common. I'd also experienced care and treatment in which small changes could not only have saved the National Health Service (NHS) money but, more importantly, would have led to significant improvements for patients.

What's it like – did you enjoy learning about co-production?

I enjoyed contributing and wanted to change things for the better. Discovering my skills in leadership, creative thinking and problem solving was energising. I could also see that the people around me in co-production teams, including those in paid employment, have their own histories and sometimes also struggle with health issues. I started to realise that overcoming adversity and living with the conditions I have has equipped me well for such work, not just with baggage. I've learnt to be more forgiving of those on the front line of services, as some of those also had been through tough times and were often just as frustrated as me with the system and processes they have to work within. In short, it's about building relationships and respecting the fact that whatever title or tag you have to your name, everyone plays an equal part in making services better and more responsive to the needs of those receiving them.

Are there any downsides to collaborative working?

It can be very isolating. I am often reminded that I am never really 'an equal'. I am not one of them. For someone who has experienced depression, this feeling of isolation carries particular risks. Negative thoughts and feelings – that I don't really fit in or belong – cause me to become hyper-vigilant to rejection, and I have to work hard to keep such thoughts and feelings in check. At times my depression will completely take me over, and I disengage from the very things I enjoy and value. I just shut myself off. I'm lucky, as most of the people I work with have got to know me well, over time and by working together, and often welcome me back into the fold. Speaking of which, this brings me to why we are using this interview technique for this chapter. My family and I have been through a lot lately, and as you know, Julie, I was going to pull out of writing this chapter. But instead of just writing me off as many have done in my past, you decided to work with me and find a way to meet my current needs, and together we have worked hard over many phone calls to nail down the true spirit of co-production. In doing so, I believe we have actually demonstrated that very thing: not giving up, always persevering and no matter how hard things have got, we – or rather, you – have stuck by me and enabled me to contribute to this book; that is true co-production!

But back to the original question: I see different rules in play as well, even in co-production teams. What I call the 'two hats' argument goes something like this: when a service user is not present, others remember their experiences of illness or treatment and move into that space, wearing what they sometimes call their 'two hats'. Their professional or manager hat seems to create no conflict with their patient or carer hat. Indeed, sometimes both sit so comfortably that it's natural to wonder why a service user is necessary to co-production at all. I want to say in response to this argument that, yes, of course, most of us, unless we are unusually fortunate, have fleeting or even significant experiences of poor health or have cared for others over the course of an adult life. We can use our memory and imagination to think about the consequences of not having resources or people to help, and we can think empathically about how we would feel and what we would need. However, this is a different kind of experience to living over time with an identity altered by a reliance on care or treatment, and often welfare; of losing people and roles and opportunities because of health problems. It is a very different experience to having become politicised by such changed prospects and by the interminable need to negotiate access to help and make sure the right words are used. Presuming to be able to speak from the service user point of view as though it is simply a hat, to be donned and doffed at will, is at best naive and at worst dismissive and invalidating of others' lived experience.

How do you reflect on your experiences?

Since the Recovery College East, I have worked on local and national projects with NHS England, shaping policy around expenses for people with disabilities, helping design training resources, and I also founded Twitter School, a virtual space for people to learn the basics of social media online. Along with Justine Thomson, who worked for NHS England at the time, we delivered training in person and followed it up online using the #TwitterSchool hashtag, as we both believe social media is an essential skill that brings many benefits leading to a more informed and connected workforce. In fact, through Twitter I formed many relationships that led me to real-world projects such as The Kings Fund. They were looking for people with lived experience of health services to work with an independent commission, which sought to advise government on the future of health and social care. Nine of us worked closely with the commissioners, who were all highly esteemed economists, led by Dame Kate Barker. Our job was to discuss from our perspective how these economic decisions would impact our individual lives on a human level, not just an economic one. After giving a well-received talk at the launch of the interim report and following it up with a blog for The Kings Fund website, I was asked to deliver other talks on leadership and my work, such as the Change Leaders programme in Newmarket. At other times, I've worked closely with my local NHS Trust, and third-sector organisations such as MIND. (See further reading at the end of the chapter.)

Things don't always go smoothly, though. My involvement with the Recovery College ended when I insisted the 'students' should have representation on the steering group and decide policy. That was what I understood the ethos of recovery to be: that we are all equals and have an equal say in how things go. But not everyone agreed, and other factors became more important than having a democratic approach to decision-making, for example smooth running and efficiency, and sustainability. I soon felt the doors closing on me, resulting in me no longer wanting any participation at all as I was very fragile at the time. At first, I took this very badly. It fed into the old feelings of previous rejections and being shunned. Over time, I picked myself up and started to push on other doors, one of which led me to 'Patient Leadership', the term first coined by Mark Doughty and David Gilbert (see, for example, Gilbert and Doughty, 2013). Both authors offer many more resources online. The tongue-in-cheek nature of the term was to challenge the stigmatising nature of the term *patient*. A patient is seen as a passive recipient of NHS services, with no value other than to be 'fixed'. It had become a very disempowering word, but still an important one, because we are patients: patients with life-changing illness, disability or experience that have been at the blunt end of services for often decades, or even a lifetime. We can repeatedly challenge this stigmatisation by saying we – patients – aren't problems to be fixed or managed, but untapped assets that the NHS could use to its advantage. However, in order for system leaders to truly recognise us as equals, then we must become recognised as leaders in our own right. Battling these life-changing circumstances has given us skills such as perseverance, courage, problem solving and, most importantly, a different way of thinking because we have all had to overcome much adversity. These are all 'leadership' skills, and when I met David and Mark, they taught me that I was more than my illness or disability; I had leadership skills – I just hadn't realised. Depression keeps you down and makes you feel useless to the world, but now I was learning more about what real leadership meant and that it wasn't about autocracy or being above other people, but about doing something different, leading by example and challenging current thinking. Change cannot happen without leadership because in order to change culture, we must put ourselves out there and show others we have a clear vision and value. In fact, by doing what I do, I give myself value and self-belief, which I didn't have before. I have a new identity of someone who knows he is a part of something bigger, a network of individuals that are doing amazing things and that, in turn, inspires others like us to see they have value too.

The term *patient leader* was new to me, and I found myself questioning how someone like me – so often feeling weak and pathetic – could even entertain the prospect of being a leader. I had many stereotypes of what that word meant. However I found myself learning more about the many meanings of leadership and about the idea that if you want change, then you must step up and be prepared to put yourself out there with clear goals, and hope others will follow your example. That's exactly what I did – with David, Mark and many others. I followed their example and learned what real leadership is all about: finding common ground, communicating your vision and repeatedly getting up when you're tackled to the ground by illness or the stubborn system you're desperately trying to change.

You specifically wanted to discuss power and how it takes different forms, shifts around between people and groups, moves things on in new ways ...

Yes. Patient leadership presents a challenge to existing power bases and hierarchies. Because of this, there are many ways in which others seek to reduce its catalytic potential. Some people find it hard to let go, to share leadership of projects, which, while no excuse, is understandable: after all, what are the implications for professionals if a service user is able to do just as well, or better, than those employed to do such work? For example, I remember being told on occasions that I was a 'volunteer', as I'm unpaid, and therefore should be doing jobs that the NHS Trust needs me to do, and that as a volunteer I must represent the Trust – in essence, be 'working for' the Trust rather than being myself working as an individual, making a contribution. Although I'm unpaid, I choose not to consider myself a volunteer, not that there is anything wrong with volunteering – it's simply a different relationship.

One way of defining a volunteer is as a helper – somebody who willingly offers his or her time and skills for free to an organisation, to carry out and further its objectives. This implies a corporate duty and loyalty and makes you, in effect, part of the system, just like a member of staff, but without the salary. It can be interpreted, as somebody once put it, as implicating and involving us in the organisational mission. It suggests too that unlike paid employees, *my* time is not money – it doesn't have a cost; there are no other things I must do with my time that are more important; my time is available to be given and taken without recompense. While others check phones and clocks, arrive late or rush off to other meetings, and quantify and prioritise their involvement in terms of competing commitments, I sit there as the only unpaid person in the room. That is not how I wish to contribute my time to an organisation. I want to seek my own agenda and 'work' – as an equal respected partner with my own views, thinking about what involvement really means and ultimately coming to a common understanding and mutual respect with others also 'working' for change and improvement for patients.

What do you mean by 'your own agenda'?

I often hear people using the word pejoratively, describing service users 'bringing their own agenda'. This is often code for 'we like how we do things already and don't want anyone interfering in *our* agenda!' I often smile to myself when I'm told this reason for not involving service users. Of course service users who get involved in co-production have an agenda. I have my agenda, and I hope everyone has an agenda – that's how power works. Why would we be involved in changing services if we had no agenda? Unfortunately, when it comes to the NHS or third-sector organisations, 'agendas' are interpreted only to mean money, whether it's money to improve a service, start a new one, consult and engage others, train people or evaluate progress rigorously. And everyone is chasing the same pot of money, so it's understandable that people get frustrated, particularly with financial cuts to services and an ongoing period of austerity – there simply isn't enough to go round. But my agenda is much more than money. All the money in the world cannot buy fairness and equality, so my agenda is to promote systems and processes that make dismissing the co-production ethos impossible. I want to see all services developed, reviewed and evaluated with strong patient involvement and leadership that is not dependent on the goodwill or whim of individuals. I want to see their contribution fairly rewarded in ways that make it possible for greater numbers to be involved and to progress into paid work roles and careers.

I understand the scepticism of many who have had to gain degrees and higher level qualifications to carry out their professional duties – it's natural that people in paid work should see patients and service users who give their time freely as a threat to maintaining essential services; a kind of cheaper substitute and a risk to future investment in professional staff. But this protective stance reflects other insecurities. It threatens innovation and sets up professionals and patient leaders in a false opposition to each other. It means that if a service user were to come up with a ground-breaking idea or project – even with support from medical professionals and well-respected research bodies – not only are they likely to be at the back of the queue, cap in hand for small amounts of money, but also under suspicion of seeking to replace or usurp paid workers. Reductions in services and reports of severe shortages in mental health provision only serve to reinforce people's mistrust and suspicion of political decisions, and in turn of more radical proposals for innovation in mental healthcare.

These concerns, while natural, miss the point that co-production is itself an ethical endeavour, underpinned by a holistic and vigorous commitment to partnership working, characterised by openness and honesty and respect for others. One of the most exciting aspects of the mental health crisis service ('The Sanctuary', a joint project between MIND and Cambridgeshire and Peterborough NHS Foundation Trust, offering a safe haven for people experiencing a mental health crisis: see Cambridgeshire and Peterborough NHS Foundation Trust, 2016) was the broad coalition of patients, third-sector organisations, managers, professionals, academics and commissioners, all sharing goals while seeing different possibilities and contributing unique perspectives. I have seen this principled commitment to collaboration reduce over time (possibly inevitably) as initiatives move from the creative phase to the more established, operational stage. Individuals take ownership and want to run things in their own way, no doubt to prove their worth (to those who pay for services, including attenders, families, commissioners and funding bodies) and to keep their service funded and running – without the more analytical, questioning stance offered by critical friends. If co-production is to become mainstream and non-negotiable, then mechanisms to embed its founding principles firmly in all aspects of practical day-to-day implementation are urgently needed. Co-production is not only a start-up activity but is part of the culture of an organisation.

So, Dominic, you keep returning to the idea of 'work' – What is so important to you about it?

Firstly, it's simple: I do not accept payment for what I do, as I have been scarred by being put through the benefits system most of my life, mainly because I've been trying to hold down a job – ironically, that means more assessments when I've lost a job through illness. Just the thought of calling DWP [the Department of Work and Pensions] fills me with dread and causes me anxiety, as I've been assessed so many times over the years. I have lost trust. Every encounter reinforces my mistrust and sets back my progress and well-being. I begin to feel as though 'they' are just looking for reasons to penalise me rather than helping me into paid work, which triggers the familiar negative thoughts and feelings of inadequacy and worthlessness. So I refuse to define 'my work' as 'work that is paid for' – instead, I define my work as the contribution I choose to make, the insights, knowledge and experience I choose to bring to a project, and the things I can achieve with other people. This way *I* have power – power and control over my own time, to give or to walk away, to speak my mind and to advocate for others who are unable to exercise power at present. I am not beholden, or indebted or 'helping' another's agenda – I am giving freely on the understanding that the gift is mine to give, not someone else's to take. I insist on payment, but I always turn it down – because it's an important principle to me that people are paid for their expertise *if they wish to be*, and if they are able to receive payment without risking other sources of income. As patients working in co-production, if we do not do this, we marginalise those who cannot afford to contribute simply because they are unable to afford to get to their hospital appointment, let alone get to a meeting with a group of people on relatively large salaries compared to those on benefits. If we only ever use 'volunteers' and offer no paid work, then that can often mean only white, older, retired individuals from a certain social class are able to afford to become engaged in co-production, in my experience. While individuals from all groups in society may be extremely talented and hold a wealth of life experience, they are not representative of our richly diverse and ever-changing society, so in the interests of all of us, we must get the balance right. I also believe, in an NHS that is increasingly privatised, we must attribute value to our expertise and time. Otherwise, we risk giving away our time not to the NHS, but to private sector profits. Besides, if we don't attribute monetary value to our expertise, then why should anyone else?

Secondly, more complex and most frustrating is the need to manage my own health. Picture this: you have a meeting at 9 a.m., 45 miles away, and you need to get there on time. Simple! Well, no, far from it. Strong antidepressants and painkillers mean that just waking and getting up, feeling fit enough to get ready and prepare for the meeting ahead and then driving a long distance is a challenge – and not an easy one. It means not only fighting the back pain once you finally wake up (antidepressants can have a hangover effect) but also recognising and overcoming the inevitable feelings of negativity that lurk, ever present (a bit like the living room full of ghosts in *Truly, Madly, Deeply*). Yes, the pills help, but they are no magic bullet, and sadly their beneficial effects all too often come hand in hand with some less welcome consequences.

So why do you put yourself through all this – do you ever think about giving up the co-production work?

Well I want to change things, but also I need a purpose, a reason to live. After many years of blocking life out on heroin and wallowing in self-pity and suicidal thoughts, I know I must keep going. It can be very hard, and it sounds self-indulgent to describe my problems, but I don't know how I can help people to understand how best to support service users to co-produce services if I'm not honest about the barriers I face just getting to a meeting on time. Also, good mental health isn't only about avoiding harms or stress – it requires certain conditions if it is to flourish. My health benefits from intellectual stimulation, from a sense of being involved in the future, of having plans and seeing milestones achieved. The self-esteem that comes from friendships and belonging, and from shared achievements, counters the negative thoughts and offers me an alternative sense of myself to reflect upon.

I want to continue to be involved in co-production because I want to be one of many, part of a pipeline of involvement, preparing and supporting others to step forward and take up training opportunities, to become patient leaders and to find stimulation and reward in the work of improving mental health provision. I put myself through it, and do my best to encourage others to persist, because I know the deck isn't always stacked fairly in life, and I want to do what I can to realise a vision for real change. For example, I want to see not one, but two or more service users on every project board, with service user involvement integrated into every aspect of organisations' governance structures. The more people involved, the more capability we produce, as we are able to step in and support one another without the stress of being the single, highly visible trailblazer. To maintain my calm and well-being, I have to know that I can dip out if my health is too poor – without feeling I have failed or succumbing to shame and negativity – and that I can step right back in again as soon as I am able. I want to make this sense of responsibility to myself – and to my family and fellow service users – normal and everyday, and in every way equal to the sense of responsibility felt towards professional colleagues and to commissioners and funders. I do not want to give up on the idea that health services, in particular the NHS, belong to all of us, and we all have a role to play in its improvement and survival.

I persevere for another important reason. After overcoming all these practical issues and health considerations, I have to navigate more insidious, less visible barriers to involvement. These revolve around the stigma attached to mental illness and the often uninformed or unhelpful perceptions of how much service users are able to achieve in co-production. I've already mentioned the reluctance of some to share leadership and the way in which power is viewed as a possession to be wrestled over rather than as a dynamic feature of relationships. Sometimes it is difficult to realise when this is happening, especially when people are skilful and gracious in their interpersonal relationships. It can be revealed in unexpected ways, sometimes when my guard is down, and seem all the more wounding in a context of general goodwill and inclusion. I was helped by the way The King's Fund talks of *collaborative leadership*, which only works if the person in the position of power is willing to share leadership. The project I worked on was unique (Barker, 2014) and again many resources are available, including my own blogs for The King's Fund (Stenning, 2014a, 2014b). The Barker Commission is something I'm very proud to have been a part of, and although not perfect, it was a bold step to work with people with lived experience and expertise. In some cases, having someone sit at the table, giving opinions based on years of accessing services, is no good at all if nobody is really listening or involving the person in a meaningful way. I have no ambition simply to be a way of ticking the 'involvement box', one of the most tokenistic and ultimately demeaning forms of patient involvement.

I had an experience recently that illustrates tokenism at its most subtle, possibly – if I am generous – unintended. After being a member of a project delivery board for more than a year, like others I was excited to learn that we were to be visited by the Secretary of State for Health. The event was to be well publicised, and our project launched in a very significant way. We planned, as a group, the board 'round table' at which the Secretary of State for Health was to be a participant, and a healthy debate took place regarding venue, scheduling and so on. I was pleased to be part of some very thoughtful and moral decisions regarding a truthful account of the project's progress and challenges. After all this, it wasn't until my invitation and the timetable for the visit arrived some days later that I understood I was not invited to the round table part of the event with the Secretary of State. Instead, my name was included in a subsequent part of the visit entitled 'meet the patients'. As happy and proud as I am to be part of a meeting with other people who use mental health services, my exclusion from the board meeting was not something I could accept. I made my feelings known to my colleagues, who rapidly reversed the decision. I was subsequently invited to the round table meeting, where I succeeded in making my contribution directly to the man himself. Indeed, I must have said something memorable, as I was asked discreetly to meet individually with the Secretary of State for Health to elaborate on my assertion that the work of the Department of Health would benefit greatly from more direct consultation with service users rather than only with the traditional hierarchy. At the time, I felt surprised and disappointed by the original plan not to include me in the round table discussion; however, it gave me great pride to find out later that many colleagues had backed my corner to be fully included in the event as an equal.

What does being treated as an equal really mean to you?

No matter how good I am at what I do, if I'm not given the opportunity to really be involved as an equal, then I simply can't do much about it other than move on to someone else willing to work with me, respecting the unique knowledge and skills I bring and the contributions I can make. Just getting out of bed each day when very depressed takes courage and perseverance. Still being on the planet shows tenacity that many in much more privileged circumstances lack. I sound confident, but it's not always like this. Getting knocked back or treated differently due to my health or diagnosis can really hurt, and getting involved in a project only to find I'm the token service user, there to enable a box to be ticked or a rubber stamp to be stamped, can really drag me down. Having confidence – or pretending to – takes a lot of work, so if those around you do not genuinely value your presence, then it can only be a matter of time before you doubt yourself again.

What of the future?

There are many admirable projects I have been involved in, and most of them have been carried out in such a way that I have been able to truly contribute and influence the ultimate delivery and implementation of our plans. I have felt respected as an equal and really listened to, and feel fortunate to have been part of each project. So there is a double-edged sword. On the one hand, to commit fully to a team and project, and to invest hope in both processes and outcomes, it is necessary to trust one's colleagues and understand how power operates in dynamic and creative ways within co-production. Hope and trust bring with them the risk of disappointment, the possibility (likelihood) of subtle forms of discrimination, and stress, both healthy and risky types. On the other hand, involvement done well, when there is a real passion to involve service users as equals, brings immeasurable benefits not just to the project's outcomes but also to all the people involved. Good communication generates and deepens empathy, and that is a powerful thing. Without understanding what people using services need (and where, when and how they need them), the project's effectiveness will be limited. Often unnecessary expenses will be incurred, mistakes and miscalculations made, efficiency inevitably decreased, and – hey, presto – the new, shiny project will cause as many problems as it solves.

We have seen a real shift in the agenda for people with life-changing illness or disability co-designing and even delivering healthcare services. I am proud to know many of them and have learnt much. Some are sadly no longer here for many reasons, not least the very health conditions that drove them to get involved in co-production. It is out of respect for their efforts, and in order to build on their achievements, that we must work harder to share leadership and to resist the polarising, if understandable, urges to hold on to the reins of power too tightly or relinquish them completely. From experience, I know it can be hard to find a middle course and trust in others, but that is what we must do if we are to survive a shrinking healthcare budget and growing demand on mental health services. It means working with third-sector organisations and individual service users and their networks, to embrace new ways of thinking. 'Engagement' by survey or focus group, cherry-picked responses and central command and control has had its day.

How can we get there?

A lack of financial investment in co-production is a significant barrier. How can we expect to work with diverse groups of service users without investing in them – in short, paying them for not only their expenses but for the hidden costs (e.g. of alternative caregiving costs) and understanding the real value of their time? Clear guidance and an appreciation of the complexities of claiming welfare benefits and working, while staying safely inside allowable parameters, is essential if people are to make informed choices. For those able to make the step away from benefits, then a fair rate of pay and a step onto the career ladder is the only acceptable way forward, with flexible arrangements to support those re-entering the workplace. Relying on retrospective settlement of expenses completely excludes those unable to spend money up front with no idea when it will be reimbursed. Commitments to support involvement in the form of hospitality, accommodation, parking arrangements and so on must not be explicit and easy to access (see, e.g., National Institute for Health Research, 2013). If we want co-production and a diversity of experience, we must be prepared to pay for it.

I often hear the argument that if we pay people, we will attract those doing it for the wrong reasons – yet I would not accuse a healthcare professional of being motivated only by money. This argument reinforces the fear that we are not valued, but merely tokens of involvement, and I find it sneaks up on me and affects my behaviours; I often censor myself from asking too many questions, as I don't want to be accused of being difficult or of holding up progress. Yet that is the essence of co-production. A recent experience illustrated the many challenges of moving into co-production as paid work. A charity asked me to do a piece of work as a team member, albeit unpaid initially, in order to secure paid work further along the project. The organisation's Human Resources Department staff were unable to configure an arrangement for me to participate in necessary ways, jeopardising the proffered future paid work. An existing employee was therefore required to undertake the preliminary work earmarked for my voluntary contribution and, in the process, assumed the very work role I had been asked to undertake later on in the project. In doing so, the fairly junior employee became the notional manager of my voluntary contribution, and in effect my superior and line manager, while depending on me to carry out the work that I know I would have done differently. Now the 'job' became an unpaid volunteer role with no prospect of the paid work opportunity in the future, as had previously been agreed.

In conclusion, what can we take away from this?

There is no 'bad person' in this scenario: bureaucracy is bureaucracy, rules are rules, and project deadlines wait for no one. It was not personal; indeed people were rooting for me and doing their best to make the situation work out. Yet I struggle with the injustice of it and with the familiar feelings of insecurity and inadequacy, wondering if I should know my place just because I'm unpaid. Then I remember *that's how power works* – and I do not want either to throw the reins away in despair or grasp them so tightly I make life impossible for those trying hard to learn new ways of co-production. So I have taken on the voluntary role (as I will take on others in the future) and fully intend to make it my own – to be a leader, to be creative and bold, and generous, and to challenge thinking until I leave a positive mark on the organisation. This is my ground-up view of co-production, and I want to contribute to this collection because I can see from my vantage point the ethical dimensions of identities forged through meaningful work, of equality expressed in fair treatment and explicit processes, and of the potential of power when it is given generously and held by many.

Thank you Dominic

References

Barker, K. (2014) A new settlement for health and social care: final report of the independent Commission on the Future of Health and Social Care in England. London: The Kings Fund. https://www.kingsfund.org.uk/sites/default/files/field/field_publication_file/Commission%20Final%20%20interactive.pdf (accessed 12 September 2017).

Cambridgeshire and Peterborough NHS Foundation Trust, news release, (2016). http://www.cpft.nhs.uk/Latest-news/Mental-health-safe-haven-opens-in-Cambridge.htm (accessed 12 September 2017).

Gilfoyle, S. and Hodge, M. Road to Recovery: our stories of hope, Recovery College East, Cambridgeshire and Peterborough NHS Foundation Trust. http://www.cpft.nhs.uk/about-us/recovery-college-east.htm (accessed 12 September 2017).

Gilbert, D. and Doughty, M. The quiet revolutionaries: patient leaders. *Health Service Journal*, 19 February 2013. https://www.hsj.co.uk/leadership/the-quiet-revolutionaries-patient-leaders/5054198.article (accessed 12 September 2017).

National Institute for Health Research (2013) INVOLVE: Values, principles and standards for public involvement in research. http://www.invo.org.uk/wp-content/uploads/2013/12/INVOLVE-Principles-and-standards-for-public-involvement-1-November-2013.pdf (accessed 12 September 2017).

Stenning, D. (2014a) It's time to start asking and answering the tough questions (blogpost). https://www.kingsfund.org.uk/blog/2014/04/its-time-start-asking-and-answering-hard-questions-view-expert-experience. (accessed 12 September 2017).

Stenning, D. (2014b) A view from experience at the Barker Commission Interim report launch. The Kings Fund. https://www.kingsfund.org.uk/audio-video/dominic-stenning-view-experience-barker-commission-interim-report-launch. (accessed 12 September 2017).

11

Ethics ... 'We do that on Fridays'

Rebecca Dunne

Introduction

As a new medical student, I was unsure for some time of the point of ethics education. The subject seemed irrelevant given how much we needed to learn in terms of medical knowledge, and viewed in this way it felt as though we used valuable time that could be better spent. Now in my final year, I understand far better why a lifelong approach to ethics education is fundamental to my medical practice. I find it much more interesting, and even in classroom settings, using more abstract examples, I am able to draw on my practical learning and experiences from clinical placements to explore ideas. I have found that it is only by coming to grips with ethical issues in practice, in what Beckett and Hager (2002, p. 23) call 'organic workplace learning', that classroom-based study begins to make sense. In this article, I reflect on aspects of my practice placements where ethical awareness and reasoning started to become central to my learning. Developing ethical sensitivity is what Rest et al. (2000) (further discussed by Bebeau, 2002) considered to be the first component of moral development, the others being judgement, motivation and commitment. I also discuss areas where I still feel unsure about my feelings with regards to medical complexities and review some of the decision-making processes I have observed and participated in. My reflections may seem somewhat straightforward or even naive to more experienced practitioners, but I am writing this chapter for fellow medical students and other novice health professionals. I hope they will find it helpful and, if they recognise some of the feelings I raise, that they may not feel so alone in their concerns.

Before beginning my postgraduate medical degree, I studied neuroscience as an undergraduate and was shocked to discover human cadavers were used for us to learn anatomy. I wondered what I had let myself in for. After my initial panic reaction, I began to think about the person who had volunteered her- or himself, or at least what remained of this person after death, for medical training or research. What I realise now is that I was thinking about the ethics of our use of cadavers to learn basic anatomy. We weren't undertaking any medical procedures or advancing research, but just doing exercises in recognition. I became aware of many issues and asked myself, did these volunteers understand their body was going to be used for anatomy education, or did they believe it would contribute to ground-breaking research such as finding a cure for cancer or at least advancing a doctor's procedural skills? I wondered whether they appreciated their mortal remains might be inspected by a group of neuroscience students who didn't really know what they were looking at, might have little serious interest in either anatomy or a future medical career, and who might possibly have learned every bit as much from some form of virtual learning. Did the question itself matter as long as, when alive, the person had freely made a decision motivated by altruism?

This is my first memory of posing ethical questions, and I can see that my interest was provoked and my awareness heightened. However, throughout my degree in medicine I have learned a great deal more about the connection between ethics and the everyday experiences of medical life. Much of our learning and teaching takes place during clinical placements, which rightly take up the majority of medical training, particularly in the latter years of study. Learning medicine is very practical, even though it is also dependent on our spending hours studying textbooks and journal articles. I consider my course to have been excellent in many ways; medical staff and others have been outstanding both with their patients and with their students, and on many occasions the more obvious 'clinical' ethical issues have been discussed openly. Yet I don't think ethical issues arising from more routine or everyday work are given as much attention in this practical context as they need to be. I have often been left to myself to think through very complex issues and practices while feeling distressed by experiences and outcomes that are intrinsically disturbing. Pauly et al. (2012) discuss the 'moral distress' of health work when personal values which conflict with work practices and feelings of helplessness are compounded by a lack of time and support to reflect and process events. One response to this is described as the development of resilience, or the ability to be 'persistent, committed, adaptable' and to seek to improve systems, taking a principled position when needed (Howe et al., 2012, p. 352); however, such a response is by no means guaranteed.

Students' experiences of ethical problems in clinical practice

Research into medical students and their ethical development is well established. Professional development and professionalism is often a focus for inquiry, with research suggesting that learning and teaching approaches, curriculum design, assessment approaches, role models and student selection are important factors (Passi et al., 2010). So I was interested to see that a study set in Australian general practice used recorded tutorials to explore the ethical and professional concerns raised by medical students (Sturman et al., 2014). Themes generated included mixed or contradictory messages in ethics teaching, predicaments reflecting status differences and boundary issues, and finally altered expectations of the general practitioners' role given the changing scope of practice (Sturman et al., 2014, p. 90). It was a rigorous study with valuable outcomes, data from tutorials interpreted and communicated by the researchers who are also medical educators. Nonetheless research conducted by three junior doctors and a medical student resonated much more directly with my own experiences. A much older study based in Toronto (Hicks et al., 2001) used surveys (completed by 103 students) followed by focus groups (with a total of 20 students). The kinds of 'ethically problematic situations' encountered by medical students were elicited and described in three categories:

➤ Students' involvement in care perceived to be substandard

➤ Responsibility beyond a student's capacities

➤ Conflict between the priorities of medical education and those of patient care. (Hicks et al., 2001, p. 709)

I have chosen to use these categories to organise my reflections on some ethically problematic situations, drawing on practical experiences. I have not related any incidents, people or situations directly; that is, I have combined and altered circumstances to ensure no individual is identified, while seeking to retain the essential issues they raise.

Perceptions of substandard care

Substandard care is clearly an area of considerable concern for the medical profession, for health professionals and managers more generally, and of course for all of us using health services as patients, caregivers, friends and families. The Mid Staffordshire Public Inquiry Report (Francis,

2013) described through patients' and carers' accounts a deeply distressing culture of failure to care, described by Quick (2014, p. 1) as one of many similar inquiries to find 'closed hierarchical systems, fear of blame and punishment, toleration of bad practices, and a failure to learn from patient and staff feedback'. In an extensive and multi-method study examining culture and behaviour in the UK's National Health Service (NHS), Dixon-Woods et al. (2013, p. 110) found substandard care, or 'dark spots', 'where staff were challenged to provide quality care, were harried or distracted, or were preoccupied with bureaucracy', and contrasted this with 'bright spots' characterised by teamwork that was caring and compassionate, cooperative and committed to learning and innovation.

'Dark spots' leading to 'substandard care' are extremely complex, especially when inadequate time or resources play a part, given that it is very rare for anyone in medical and health professions to want to deliberately harm someone in any way. For medical students, substandard care is something that can be upsetting and perhaps also something they have little control over. I am reminded of the case where Victoria Fearne, a 25-year-old medical student, tried to prevent two surgeons from removing a patient's only healthy kidney by mistake (Alleyne, 2002), but as a medical student she was dismissed as 'wrong', and the surgeons continued to remove the incorrect kidney. Many staff may at times be subject to the hierarchies that exist, with negative consequences. In another example, during the course of a routine procedure, nurses watched surgeons and anaesthetists work hard – incorrectly and ultimately unsuccessfully – to save the life of Elaine Bromiley, knowing there was a correct course of action that was not being followed, yet not quite assertive or powerful enough in their attempts to intervene (Harmer, 2005). Since these cases, actions have been taken to improve such areas of care. However, I feel there is still a sense of hierarchy within medicine that can make it difficult to raise concerns to seniors. For certain situations, had I been given them as a case study on a piece of paper in a classroom, I would have known exactly what to do – I would have anticipated that I would have done 'the right thing'.

However the following (composite) scenario demonstrates this is easier said than done:

> You are a medical student. You are on a ward round with the consultant and junior doctor. The patient has a cardiac arrest in front of you. You have never witnessed a cardiac arrest before, and the junior doctor is inexperienced in dealing with this situation. The consultant begins cardiopulmonary resuscitation (CPR). You can see his technique is outdated and does not adhere to the most recent CPR training you received two months ago but have never

performed yourself. Nurses arrive to help with CPR and crowd around watching the consultant as he continues. No one is intervening.

What do you do?

In my own head I have an ideal imagined situation: I politely vocalise my concerns over the consultant's technique and ask if he minds letting someone more recently trained in CPR take over and allow for best patient care. In an ethics class, this response might get you a gold star.

It might be a good approach; however, in real life and with a bit more thought, it becomes so much more difficult. Within this scene lies an ethical dilemma with alternative courses of action to be weighed each against the other – intervening when aware of an incorrect or poor standard of care being administered versus allowing a colleague who has embarked on a course of action to follow through. Is standing by simply wrong – a collective mistake? Or are there ethical arguments *against* intervening as well as in support of it? An argument based on the consequences of acting or not acting might include a calculation of the differential benefits of the older technique compared with the newer technique. It might factor in the relative skills of individuals and question whether a (potentially) more practised/confident application of an older technique might be as good or better in terms of outcome than a (possibly) novice application of a newer and better technique, raising questions of the relative skill and experience of the observers on the ward. Such a consequentialist calculation would surely factor in the patient's age and health condition, the speed of administering CPR versus seconds or minutes lost in discussion or negotiation, and include evidence of likely outcomes. An ethical defence of *not* intervening, or of the consultant's actions, based on consequences, would seem at least to be possible in theoretical terms and would be part of a critical incident analysis into such an event.

If the principled approach (Gillon, 1985) dictates doing the best for the patient in the moment regardless of these unknown (probably unknowable) comparable outcomes, we might agree that the most up-to-date, evidence-based approach to CPR is likely to be 'best'. The classroom-based response – that this is a straightforward decision – reflects such a clear and unambiguous approach yet may not 'stick' or lead to action in the scenario outlined. Virtue ethics (MacKenzie, 2009) might prompt a reflection on what being a good doctor, in that particular place and time, would mean. Among the staff in the scenario, were there particular factors contributing to collective inaction – such things as place, resources, preceding events, beliefs and so on, and on relationships? For example was there a strong sense of team loyalty or friendly collegiality, or dominance, or too rigid a hierarchy? Might this be what Dixon-Woods et al. (2014) would identify as a 'dark spot'? As a textbook scenario, it is impossible to know all the complexities, even to judge 'right' or 'wrong'. Only the lived experience can inform how people do, or should, act. Sometimes what seems straightforward when presented as an ethical dilemma in a theoretical sense needs to be played out in practice as a medical or team decision if its complexity is to be appreciated. However, what is important is that inaction is not considered the norm. But I do recognise also how novices may question their own suitability for medicine or doubt their judgement skills, or even try to fit in, rather than understanding the importance of culture and leadership (Satterwhite et al., 2000).

Ethical decisions make almost as great a part of our job as medical decisions, yet Brooks and Bell (2017) found in a survey of lead academics that, despite the national core curriculum for ethics and law in UK medical schools (GMC, 2015), the extent to which this is implemented varies across medical schools. Although all respondents (11 out of a possible 33) felt students were well prepared for ethical practice, seven reported that ethics is not included in clinical placement learning objectives (Brooks and Bell, 2017). Citing a lack of time and suitable placements, the authors conclude that not all doctors are adequately prepared for ethical decision-making in clinical practice. Following my student experience, I found myself asking: in some practice settings, is a good moral compass expected to suffice?

In keeping with a moral compass, it is a doctor's desire (as well as duty) to 'save' people – it is our job; we feel like we have failed if we do not. But is this always an ethical stance? I have been taught that resuscitation is not always the correct or ethical course of action. I appreciate that there are, of course, challenging ethical issues surrounding a lack of resuscitation, and chance of survival/quality of life versus a peaceful death is at times a well-nigh impossible judgement. Medicine, especially in elderly care, is evolving so that consideration of 'quality of life' may outweigh 'life' itself. But how quickly can we as doctors adapt to advances in what should be considered 'right' and 'wrong' – or best for the patient in a particular set of imperfect and fast-changing circumstances – and how much is our 'gut instinct' competing with our more rational decision-making processes? Although ethical frameworks explored and debated in the (ideally) safe and trusting atmosphere of the classroom are helpful, as professionals and as humans it is very difficult when physically, emotionally and intellectually involved in a clinical crisis requiring swift action. This topic is deeply and thoughtfully discussed by Caldwell (2015), who, in a letter to the *British Medical Journal* (BMJ), concludes that a defensive and risk-averse approach to CPR is threatening the best interests of patients and the likelihood of 'ordinary deaths'.

Responsibility beyond capacity

On the one hand, much of what I did on placement during my time at medical school could be seen as having responsibility beyond my capability; on the other hand, I see it all as an essential and realistic part of my development. As a doctor, you continue to learn and will face things that you do not know how to do or how to respond to throughout your career. However, as a student I know I did not always manage the limits of my competence particularly well. For example, when a patient asked me something like: 'Is this the first time you've done this procedure?' I did not know what to say. It has been suggested to us that we might reply: 'I've practised it many times, don't worry'. However, is it ethical to say this when the truth is, I have practised it only in a simulated environment, never with a human being? I have come to think that how to respond may depend on the patient in front of me: ethics, I feel, should not be 'one size fits all' but should be sensitive to the context and needs of the patient, insofar as these are possible to assess.

When I saw a cyclist knocked off his bicycle by a van at a roundabout. I immediately thought that it should be my responsibility to go and see if he was badly hurt, but I felt unprepared and scared. Since then, whenever I drive somewhere after a day's work at the hospital, I always want to remove my 'medical student' lanyard in case there is an accident on the road. I do not want someone to see that I am a medical student and therefore expect me to help and to know what to do. I ask myself: is that unethical? It's not that I would not want to help, but that I would be worried I am not experienced enough as a student to know what to do, so I avoid that potential situation. I do now appreciate, however, that, as a doctor, medicine and ethics encompass every part of our lives, every minute of the day, in a way that I had not fully recognised and cannot seek to avoid.

Conflict between the priorities of medical education and those of patient care

Having been introduced to the use of cadavers as a neuroscience undergraduate, solely for the purpose of learning anatomy, during medical school we used manikins to learn some basic clinical techniques. This is an excellent way of learning, as a starting point, coming to understand all the possible technicalities and difficulties, in the sure knowledge that the patient-manikin cannot come to harm. But it is also in a sense meaningless because of this difference. Taking blood from a real person is far more difficult and complex. It is about the procedure itself, but also about the person whose blood is being taken. In some ways, this is the difference between ethics in the classroom, which often seems relatively straightforward when discussed in the abstract, and ethics in practice – which takes on a different meaning when faced with relationships, pain, emotion, and life or death implications.

The conflict between medical learning and patient care also arose on an occasion when I had tried to put a cannula into an older patient, but failed. In these circumstances, I would normally have asked a doctor to take over. However, I tried a second time, as the patient was passive and not displaying discomfort. Afterwards, I asked myself the question: 'Was repeated cannulation wrong in this instance?' I recognise now that my thinking was naive in different ways. First of all, I was not confident of the man's ability to give informed consent. Because the immediate need was to take blood, I concentrated on 'learning' the task required of me, trying harder after the first failed attempt. Secondly, I responded differently to my unsuccessful attempt, changing my normal practice, not realising the patient's vulnerability ought to have acted as a prompt for greater attention to good process, not less. On another occasion, I was taking blood from a patient already assessed to be difficult to take blood from. I failed twice, yet she encouraged me to keep trying until I succeeded. She had given me her consent, and I could see no reason not to continue, but the junior doctor I was working with intervened. She told the patient firmly that she was not a pincushion and that I couldn't possibly keep taking blood from her. I had interpreted consent superficially without considering the implications or the disposition of the patient; until my colleague reminded us both that such 'practice' was not appropriate.

Obviously, both these scenarios are problematic to reflect upon, and I learned a good deal about myself and about ethical practice through doing so. Both presented learning opportunities, but not, as I had expected, of the technical or practical type. I learned that while I could 'practise' my technique – and become better at cannulating or taking blood in the future, even possibly saving someone's life in an emergency – in doing so I would be abusing a trust and using a person as a means to my learning rather than respecting her as an end in herself. Learning about different ethical theories in a classroom relies on analysis and debate, and the weighing up and comparison of different possible courses of action. However, when making a treatment decision with a patient in front of you, very often there has to be a single response, often swiftly enacted. We cannot afford *not* to discuss and reflect on our actions in practice, where considerations can seem very different. Ethics education in practice might usefully take account of the aftermath of an intervention, as well as the analysis of factors leading to a decision. Doing so would require an openness and honesty that might be seen to contradict the need to convey confidence and professionalism, particularly given the need to pass assessments and to be trusted by patients and colleagues to undertake difficult and often new clinical interventions. Reason (2000) discusses the longer-term implications of a medical culture in which mistakes cannot be honestly reflected upon and discussed, advocating for open-learning organisational and professional environments. The aforementioned case with the surgeons' dismissal of Victoria Fearne's observation of which kidney to be removed, illustrates the very culture Reason (2000) warns us against.

So reflecting upon the everyday experiences of learning, and balancing my own needs with those of my patients, has offered important insights into ethical practice. The experiences also offer important learning about consent – including the principles underpinning genuinely informed consent, the legal framework supporting consent and the conditions necessary for promoting relationships of openness and trust to name a few – yet in the moment my own understanding of 'learning' was centred on the complicated practical tasks ahead of me. Medical students being assessed in practice are directed, by learning outcomes and assessments, to the skills and knowledge they have to demonstrate to pass and to demonstrate competence. As Brooks and Bell (2017) suggest, a greater emphasis on ethics in daily, practical clinical work would focus students' attention on the potential to learn with and from our patients, their carers and families, and our colleagues.

Reflection

Reflecting on ethical practice leads me to consider conflict in medical work more generally, and in particular between patient care and the patients' best interests. This, I believe, is one of the most complex areas of all with regard to both ethical behaviour and the relation of ethics to my personal feelings. I continue to reflect on two troubling experiences, again somewhat altered to respect privacy. In the first, a patient underwent an operation, which, through no fault of the surgeons, had not gone to plan. With a poor outcome and poor quality of life, she expressed the desire to leave hospital and to end her life. Her suicidal expressions led to her being assessed as at serious risk and being kept in hospital to prevent her attempting or possibly succeeding in taking her life. Although I appreciate that we must choose to put saving lives above everything, I still ask myself: who knows what is in someone else's best interests when the future is so uncertain, or frankly bleak? Does not wanting to live denote mental illness? Or is it a rational response to a particular diagnosis? Was our responsibility not to organise rapid community care and a discharge package that respected her wishes, rather than to take away her autonomy and legal right to refuse treatment by making another kind of diagnosis? I appreciate that my experience may have been unique and that the complexities are great. I fully understand my responsibilities as a doctor and realise this is a controversial area, but I empathised with the patient and believe that we need to keep revisiting such difficult areas, to keep discussing them, and that these are matters for national debate as well as for doctors. Especially as a student, it seems important that we are encouraged to debate and challenge the status quo.

The second situation I want to consider involves patients with a debilitating condition who opt to be treated with a new 'wonder drug'. This drug is thought of as a 'poisoned chalice' by many patients and doctors, for it revolutionises a patient's life for an indeterminate amount of time until it turns to poison and causes a progressive multifocal leukoencephalopathy (PML) – a severely debilitating (often fatal) outcome. I found myself thinking: how can we ask people desperate for symptom relief to make an informed, long-term treatment decision? Are we in fact offering a sort of 'magical' short-term cure, knowing it comes with the risk of a much worse condition in the future? I may be thinking in paternalistic ways, so properly criticised by people who want to be fully involved in their treatment decisions. The information on this particular intervention is difficult to interpret even with medical knowledge (NICE, 2007), so it is questionable whether an informed decision in the absence of such understanding is possible. This dilemma is similar to new treatments for many different disorders, when almost impossible decisions have to be made between a known current state and an unknown future state, or between using resources on a traditional treatment or investing in a new less well-tested therapy. Patients and their families and carers will have forms of knowledge unavailable to their healthcare team, and vice versa. Calculations will be made routinely on imperfect and provisional information, risks possibly underplayed or overplayed, best guesses made in the patients' 'best interests' or by patients in desperation. Ethical practice would seem to require as much openness as possible to share uncertainties and possibilities; time for patients, professionals and others to discuss all possible outcomes and to change minds and direction; and relationships of trust that enable best interests (that may not be restricted to an individual but may include those they care about) to be discussed, reflected upon and explored fully.

In conclusion: what of the future?

One of the complexities I have begun to understand in thinking through these experiences is that there may be no precisely 'right' or 'wrong' answers in many clinical situations. Yes, as students we fully understand that we must preserve life, but this is not necessarily a straightforward process or one without its ethical problems. Sometimes distinguishing between what I would *want* to do, because I am a kind and thoughtful person, and what actually I *should* do, as an ethical professional, is testing. Working out the 'right thing to do' is not always easy – or indeed possible. My feeling is that decision-making in modern medicine may well be more difficult than ever before.

It has been claimed that 'medical students and junior doctors look for humanistic qualities – such as respect for patients and their families, compassion, honesty and integrity – in their positive role models, and that role models have an important function in the moral and professional development of medical trainees' (Sokol, 2007). I consider this to be very true, and it is important that this is heeded within a medical student's degree programme and that more time and effort is put in to discussion of the dilemmas we experience as we go through our course as novices learning and being assessed, which may be different to those encountered by practitioners and others with more experience. I also hope that some of the dilemmas that I am currently struggling with will be rehearsed with thoughtful role models during my junior doctor years. I appreciate that some of the issues I discuss here are of deep significance, and universal in nature, while others are unique and situated, and may arise from my personal naivety or lack of experience. But to me these are just as important, and having opportunities to talk about them should be part of the degree programme. This might take place in practice with the people we are working with, although time and opportunity are always going to be a problem. Reason's (2000) approach to an open culture sees mistakes as learning opportunities and is supported by the human factors, quality and safety work of Dixon-Woods (2014) and others. Learning about ethics in practice, then, whether through mistakes, near-misses or the incidents that cause moral distress, and equally through successes, is essential if a lifelong habit of reflecting and reasoning through the ethical components of situations is to be inculcated in students.

Although thinking in the abstract about moral problems is very different to acting in imperfect and uncertain circumstances, the immediacy and intensity of experiential learning offers a way in to more abstract and theoretical reasoning. Learning about, say, the Four Principles approach (Gillon, 1985) in the classroom may be enjoyable and interesting, but such ideas are less easy to make sense of in practice when knowing what to do to benefit the patient is part of the problem, or what course of action will cause least harm, much less how to respond when principles conflict. This is not to suggest a theoretical framework is meaningless – a single principle such as not doing harm, applied thoughtfully to a particular situation, can feel like a life raft at times – but, in my opinion, any given approach can only work as a starting point for exploration. Real life is untidy. I do not want to be perceived as unprofessional for criticising our everyday practices, but I am beginning to see that a framework does not, and cannot, cover every complex situation and is open to multiple interpretations in the busy, overworked, practical world of healthcare.

Most important of all, the ethical concerns I have discussed and many other similar issues impacted on my learning because I was involved with the lives and deaths and illnesses of people who deserved the highest standard of care and treatment, and I could see the impact of the decisions that I, as well as my colleagues, made. I do not think that ethics can just be 'picked up' with no explicit teaching, but I feel strongly that the relationship between learning in practical situations and learning in the classroom needs to be a much more joined-up and continuous process. I am learning that it is the conversation that surrounds practice that is important and that helps students to understand differing rationales and perspectives. Classroom teaching offers a reflective and discursive space, and – ideally – trusting and open relationships with peers, to draw together the mixture of theoretical and practical clinical work. Beginning with students' experiences and pressing concerns may offer a way into more philosophical ideas, which in turn become more meaningful when their usefulness is discovered. Classroom learning might usefully offer space and time for the expression and rehearsal of ideas; and of words and actions; and of assertiveness, diplomacy and respect that ethical practice demands of us. It is easy to imagine then how 'scaling up' debate from a single personal experience to a more intractable or high-profile dilemma, which all too often seems to involve numerous interested parties and have only unsatisfactory compromises as outcomes, may be easier when ideas have been experimented with in familiar and more routine situations. I now believe firmly that to 'do ethics on Fridays' – by which I mean in ways that separate the practical and the abstract, or at set times rather than as part of practical work, properly intertwined with relationships, places and decisions – encourages and even reinforces in students' minds its distinctness from medicine as practised. It is the experience of real people in real contexts – whether staff or patient or manager or family member – and the often intricate and difficult decisions, sometimes made under extreme pressure, that offer ethical training and preparation for future professionals. This is what has provided me with the understanding that ethics underpins all of medical practice; it is fundamental, and sometimes very scary.

References

Alleyne, R. (2002) 'Wrong kidney' surgeon ignored me, says student. *Telegraph*, 19 June 2002.

Bebeau, M.J. (2002) The defining issues test and the four component model: contributions to professional education. *Journal of Moral Education*, 31(3), pp. 271–95.

Brooks, L. and Bell, D. (2017) Teaching, learning and assessment of medical ethics at the UK medical schools. *Journal of Medical Ethics*, 43, pp. 606–12.

Beckett, D. and Hager, P. (2002) *Life, Work and Learning: Practice in Postmodernity*. London: Routledge.

Caldwell, G. (2015) *British Medical Journal* (letters), 351, p. h3769.

Dixon-Woods, M., Baker, R., Charles, K., Dawson, J., Jerzembek, G., Martin, G., McCarthy, I. et al. (2014) Culture and behaviour in the English National Health Service: overview of lessons from a large multimethod study. *British Medical Journal Quality and Safety*, 23, pp. 106–15.

Francis, R. (2013) *Report of the Mid Staffordshire NHS Foundation Trust Public Inquiry*. London: The Stationery office.

Gillon, R. (1985) *Philosophical Medical Ethics*. Chichester: Wiley.

GMC (2015) Promoting excellence: standards for medical education and training. http://www.gmcuk.org/Promoting_excellence_standards_for_medical_education_and_training_0715.pdf_61939165.pdf (accessed 12 September 2017).

Harmer, M. (2005) Independent review on the care given to Mrs Elaine Bromiley on 29 March 2005. http://www.chfg.org/wp-content/uploads/2010/11/Elaine-BromileyAnonymousReport.pdf (accessed 12 September 2017).

Hicks, L.K., Lin, Y., Robertson, D.W., Robinson, D.L. and Woodrow, S.I. (2001) Understanding the clinical dilemmas that shape medical students' ethical development: questionnaire survey and focus group study. *British Medical Journal*, 322, p. 709.

Howe, A., Smajdor, A. and Stockl, A. (2012) Towards an understanding of resilience and its relevance to medical training. *Medical Education*, 46, pp. 349–56.

Johnston, C. and Haughton, P. (2007) Medical students' perceptions of their ethics teaching. *Journal of Medical Ethics*, 33(7), pp. 418–22.

MacKenzie, C.R. (2009) What would a good doctor do? Reflections on the ethics of medicine. *HSS Journal*, 5(2), pp. 196–99.

NICE (2007) Natalizumab for the treatment of adults with highly active relapsing–remitting multiple sclerosis. https://www.nice.org.uk/guidance/ta127 (accessed 12 September 2017).

Pauly, B.M., Varcoe, C. and Storch, J. (2012) Framing the issues: moral distress in health care. *HEC Forum*, 24(1), pp. 1–11.

Passi, V., Doug, M., Peile, E., Thistlethwaite, J. and Johnson, N. (2010) Developing medical professionalism in future doctors: a systematic review. *International Journal of Medical Education*, 1, pp. 19–29.

Quick, O. (2014) Regulating and legislating patient safety: the case for candour. *British Medical Journal Quality and Safety*, (23), pp. 614–18.

Reason, J. (2000) Human error: models and management. *British Medical Journal*, 320(7237), pp. 768–70.

Rest, J.R., Narvaez, D., Thoma, S.J. and Bebeau, M.J. (2000) A neo-Kohlbergian approach to morality research. *Journal of Moral Education*, 29(4), pp. 381–95.

Satterwhite, R.C., Satterwhite, W.M. and Enarson, C. (2000) An ethical paradox: the effect of unethical conduct on medical students' values. *Journal of Medical Ethics*, 26(6), pp. 462–65.

Sokol, D.K. (2007) William Osler and the jubjub of ethics: or how to teach medical ethics in the 21st century. *Journal of the Royal Society of Medicine*, 100, pp. 544–48.

Sturman, N., Farley, R. and Jennings, W. (2014) Exploring medical student experiences of ethical issues and professionalism in Australian general practice. *International Journal of Practice-based Learning in Health and Social Care*, 2, pp. 88–95.

12

Reflections on new voices

Tula Brannelly

Discussion

In this section of the collection, three diverse chapters have a central thread on 'the real' as an aspect of practice, research and education. Hogue and Ennis-O'Connor are survivor bloggers who have shared their experiences online. They ask who has the right to use their information; as public as it is, it also belongs to them. Stenning discusses with Wintrup the challenges of offering experience to inform and transform practice, highlighting very practical changes and deeply philosophical issues as they do so. Dunne's reflection on learning and implementing ethics as a new practitioner contrasts learning about abstract ideas, with the kind of deeply personal learning acquired in and required by practical health-care work. She takes us through the ways in which she has tried to think through it to work ethically, going on to suggest that the discomforting moral questions faced by medical students offer a way into connecting with more philosophical problems.

Rebecca Hogue and Marie Ennis-O'Connor are bloggers who contribute to a world where talking about experience of illness aims to help others going through similar troubles. They point out that writing about the experience may be inward or outward facing. It may primarily be intended to help others, sharing those experiences to help others come to understand what to expect when faced by daunting assessments and treatments. Or it may be as a therapeutic self-intervention to come to terms with and understand the impacts and necessary transitions and to log the emotional aspects of illness, becoming available in time for family members to access what cannot be spoken about. They discuss who has right of access to use their personal stories. Considering Brown's chapter, where the inclusion of personal stories is seen as a way of strengthening ethics education, albeit somewhat problematically, it

is understandable how tempting these blogs are to educators, researchers and clinicians as easily accessible versions of user involvement, or as
accounts of lived experience, or even as 'data'. They offer manageable,
formed and depersonalised insights, selected and framed by someone
unlikely to have any personal knowledge or involvement in the bloggers' lives. This is an alternative to inviting people into the classroom,
who may be unpredictable, possibly emotional and, as we see in Stenning's words, most likely to bring with them an 'agenda'. Because
the personal account or conversational exchange in a blog is online, it
is easy to decide it does not immediately require relational care. But
does it? As the potential for researchers to access forms of social media
seems boundless, and as other technological advances are hailed as a
new democratisation of participation, Hogue and Ennis-O'Connor challenge conventional research ethics to find a way of acknowledging and
respecting ownership. As participators in the creation of these new
forms of data, and as creators of new types of networks, they assert that
democratising research can be achieved, but only through their willingness and that of fellow bloggers to create the new ethical processes
and permissions – possibly technological in nature – that are required.
New ways of practising care and reciprocity in research are required to
ensure that bloggers themselves, the owners of this data, are consulted
and involved in how it is used, if their considerable creative skill and generous sharing of experience is to remain freely available to others.

The ethical dimensions of service user involvement and co-production
are the focus of the chapter by Dominic Stenning and Julie Wintrup, who
discuss being involved in co-production. Their conversation throws up
some very interesting questions about how the potential for transformation can be thwarted, knowingly or otherwise. Transformation requires
power sharing for real change, and this chapter highlights the ways in
which co-production is co-opted and unethically used to support dominant hegemonic agendas. Redolent again of Brown, Stenning observes
how service users are often asked to reflect on their experience as if it is
concluded; yet he continues to be in the middle of it, working things out.
He reminds us that people with experience do not have answers readily
packaged for removal and application, a 'fix'. Reflexivity and dynamism
are intrinsic to the work Stenning describes, a willingness to *not* know
all the answers, but to work together as simultaneously vulnerable and
resilient. Although we are all cared for and carers of others, when we
are reliant or dependent or impaired, there is a need to understand the
courage and dedication it takes to get up every day and make it to the
meeting – and to make the necessary adjustments to enable people *not*
to have to travel 45 miles for a 9:00 a.m. start. Ethical practice that could
inform transformation requires professionals to realise and to diminish

their dominance, to work in solidarity with service users for change. The chapter spells out what is required for radical change in service provision, if the humanising of services often recognised as absent is to become more than rhetoric.

In her chapter, Rebecca Dunne reflects on her own experiences of coming to understand her growing awareness of ethical issues in the everyday work of healthcare. She describes how ethics is part of both practical and classroom-based learning, and goes on to share some of her doubts and uncertainties. She considers how 'live' practice differs from classroom discussions of scenarios provided to make students consider specific ways of thinking about ethics that, following experience, seem somewhat manufactured and unsatisfactory. This is a frequent discussion in ethics education – how to access the real complexity without the full knowledge of the situation under discussion and how to be able to meaningfully explore and consider the right thing to do, or even to fully appreciate the nature of a particular dilemma and its different meanings to those involved. Dunne touches on the difficulty of trying to 'apply' ethical 'rules', which can conflict. Students may experience such an approach as the need to choose between competing ethical principles, rather than as prompts for deeper thought, or ways into assessing more rigorously a situation in all of its messy context. Treated as rules, such notions as preserving life or respecting another's wishes often come into conflict, suggesting different paths and causing Dunne to wrestle with how best to apply knowledge in practice when unexpected and extraordinary events prompt the need to decide and take action in the moment, with little time to weigh alternatives. The chapter also highlights that ethical education often does not ask novice practitioners to identify what *they* think are ethical issues in practice and to bring these for discussion in the classroom. Novice practitioners have 'fresh eyes' which view the culturally embedded world differently to those who have worked through and accepted cultural practices and established norms. These fresh eyes identify the quirks and unthinkable decisions that practitioners have to make, with emotional labour and difficult questions that may be asked. There are also times when society's understanding of certain issues changes and periods where the response to those changes is negotiated through professional discourses, perhaps pioneered through education. One current example of this is the medical community's response to assisted dying and the questions this raises with the medical oath and challenges to ethical practice. It will be the new practitioners who forge the future. Dunne questions the use of powers under the mental health act and when it is right to withdraw treatment. Personal values that influence these decisions are positioned as secondary to professional practice; however, raising their status may be the only way to open up discussions that enable best practice in the best interests of patients, having those 'real' conversations. Dunne highlights how medical professionals struggle with decisions that would be better decisions if the people whom they affect were more actively involved, reminding us of Stenning's experiences of simply being omitted from decisions for no apparent reason. Including service users and patients in ethics education enables more meaningful conversations to start early in the career of practitioners, and as we are reminded by Brown, and by Hogue and Ennis-O'Connor, there are ways to do so that embed respect and adjustment into processes and relationships.

Authors of all three chapters accompany 'the real' with the emotional, the personal and the political. The consequences of these issues run deep in the practices and everyday experiences of ethical health and social care. Greater connectedness between the personal and political can only strengthen ethical practice because it humanises us all. We all know when we have received good care and when we give it; we know when we are compromised and do not have capacity. The language needed to discuss these issues is not contained in ethical codes and it does not inhabit 'rules'; it is in the everyday language of our experiences. Ethics is present in the everyday, and these chapters help us think about how to work ethically with experience.

Welcome to Paradise [1,2]

Molly Case

4th of November, 2012

06.10   Wake up 20 minutes before the alarm, nervous about new placement in a nursing home.

06.15   Have tea and cereal. The milk looks grey in the curtainy gloom.

06.30   Slip into scratchy uniform and tight trousers, fix all bits: fob watch, badge, lanyard, pens, torch.

06.45   Brush teeth, put make-up on, leave. Still nervous.

07.30   Park up the road and make my way to the nursing home. It's raining; the dockyard chimneys shine like wet clay against the sky. A boarded-up house has 'Welcome to Paradise' graffitied on the door.

07.35   Sign in at the desk, and ask for the manager. She won't be here until nine. Sit and read *The Shining*.

Tough old world, baby. If you're not bolted together tightly, you're gonna shake, rattle, and roll before you turn 30.

I'm always early. I stare at the stuffed scarecrow sitting opposite me. A sign reading *Well Meadows Care Home* hangs around its neck. It has stitched buttons for eyes.

07.50   Make my way to the first floor.

07.53   Find another human being wandering the corridors. Introduce myself. She says, 'Go and sit somewhere. The manager won't be here until nine.'

08.00   Go and sit somewhere. Continue reading *The Shining*.

Sometimes human places, create inhuman monsters.

---

[1] This shift felt like it never ended. I wanted to replicate the feeling I had in my years as a student nurse on this placement, the clock ticking, but nothing really happening; the vulnerability I felt as a student nurse, wanting to be helpful, wanting to learn and work hard, but coming up against an ingrained negative and unchanging culture. It's a tough journey being a student nurse, and I always want to remember that. MC.

[2] *Nursing the Nation and Welcome to Paradise* © Molly Case 2015; used with permission of Burning Eye Books.

08.14   Handover. Two nurses arrive in the room; neither looks at me. Turn the page.

08.30   Handover is finished. Nurse A says, 'You might as well come with me now.' I try to read her name badge.

08.40   Am piled up with towels, pads and clean clothes and sent into room 4: lovely room with all the service user's belongings inside. Feel like I shouldn't be here like this.

08.42   Nurse A says, 'You will help me wash this man. What's your name again?'

'Molly.'

08.43   Assist Nurse A with washing and dressing the service user. Chat to him about wartime in Germany and about Lancashire, where they make the towels he uses. They're the softest in England. Start feeling a bit better.

09.15   Two carers are in the lounge; more service users arrive for breakfast. I stand there seeing what needs to be done.

09.17   Grab a blue apron and start pouring tea.

'He doesn't have tea, he has coffee,' says a carer.

Put teapot down and stand and watch.

Serve porridge.

Help a lady eat her breakfast.

09.30   Sit with service users; watch *Jeremy Kyle* and *This Morning*.

10.30   Read the *Daily Mail* – nasty headlines.

11.05   Talk to a service user about her dog back home, but speak quietly as everybody is asleep.

11.10   Read the noticeboard, walk up the corridor, wonder when the manager will get here. Wish somebody would talk to me. Look for the toilets.

11.30   Manager arrives, all in red.

'I'm Jane.'

'Hello, I'm Molly.'

'You've settled in well.'

'I'm okay. I'm just helping some of the service users.'

'Good. It's good to get involved. You must get involved.'

'Okay.'

11.35   The service users are asleep. Ask the carer if we should do any activities. 'Not until three o'clock.' Watch a John Wayne film.

The technicolour looks beautiful. Brown mountains, a river raging white.

12.40   I contact another student on my phone. Can't wait to hear from her. She has the same placement.

Are you here at Well Meadow Nursing Home? Please tell me how you're finding it – feels like nobody knows I'm even here yet! Scared! xx

12.43   Knock on the office door. Nurse A looks up.

'Hi, I just wondered whether you are my mentor?'

'No, no more students. I already have two. I don't know about any more.'

'Should I ask the manager?'

No answer. Looks back to the screen.

12.45   Decide to find manager and ask about mentorship and my shifts.

12.48   Knock-knock.

'Did you want to see me?'

'Not really.'

'Maybe about who I'm working with or my rota?'

'It's Nurse A upstairs; she is your mentor.'

'Oh, I don't think she's aware of that …'

'She is. We will work out your rota later.'

'Would you mind coming upstairs with me and just checking she's okay with it?'

12.55   Stand in the office upstairs. Nurse A and manager sit at desk.

'She is your new student.'

Points at me.

'No, I already have two. No more.'

Puts her head in her hands.

'I don't want more students. I don't like students.'

'She is yours.'

'Excuse me,' I say. 'I'm sorry but I don't think this lady wants to mentor me. I don't feel comfortable in here …'

'She will mentor you.'

'Okay.'

Manager leaves.

Nurse A starts typing.

13.00　　Read the noticeboard again.

13.07　　Lunchtime. Help a service user to eat, and we chat about why we eat fish and chips on Fridays.

14.30　　Nurse A, my mentor, brings the drug trolley out.

　　　　'Should I shadow you whilst you do medication?'

　　　　'No.'

15.00　　Service users go downstairs for activities.

　　　　Ask carer whether I should attend too.

　　　　'You better stay up here with your mentor, just in case ...'

15.05　　Ask Nurse A whether she would like me to help her with anything in the office.

　　　　'It depends on what you want to learn.'

　　　　'What are you doing at the moment?'

　　　　'Care plan.'

　　　　'Can I have a look at some?'

　　　　No answer.

　　　　I sit and read some care plans.

16.00　　Nurses' meeting downstairs: they talk about a service user drinking too much Coke and two service users arguing whether *Emmerdale* should have the subtitles on or not. The room is hot with breath. Wish I could open the window. They mention a service user with swollen legs who says she wants to die. They discuss footstools. Want to ask them to talk more about her fears and anxieties.

16.15　　Another nurse mentions one of the service users has a grade two pressure sore.

　　　　'But it was grade one on Monday,' Nurse B says.

　　　　The room looks shocked.

　　　　A first-year student reported this pressure area on Monday.

　　　　Feel very sorry for the service user with the pressure sore.

16.58　　Receive a message on my phone:

　　　　It's awful! They don't want us there. What are we going to do? When I try and help, Nurse B says I'm working above my ability, and when I don't, she says I'm lazy! xx

　　　　Me: *I'm so happy to hear from you, just glad there's somebody else here! xx*

17.00　　Teatime. I help to feed a service user. Mash potato in soup.

17.46   Look at the clock.

18.00   Pass the clinical room where Nurses B and C are. Nurse B is shouting, 'They are useless, these students.' I look in at them as I pass. She shouts 'USELESS' at me and pretends to spit on the floor. Keep walking. Sit on the toilet and wonder whether that actually happened.

18.05   Wish I could go home. Think about all the people I love and who love me and feel a bit better. This is temporary. Three more weeks, just three weeks ...

18.06   Take paracetamol for a headache. Leave the toilets.

18.20   A man asks to go to his room. I offer to take him and to give him a hand with anything he needs before bed. A carer comes and takes over. 'Thanks anyway,' she says.

18.24   Sit on a footstool and watch the ITV news.

19.00   Watch *Emmerdale*.

19.30   Watch *Eastenders*. It's rubbish. It's always rubbish.

19.58   Let home early. Take the opportunity. The air outside feels great; clean after rain.

20.00   Get in the car. Welcome to Paradise.

Afterword and Acknowledgements

Julie Wintrup

I want to draw this collection to a close simply by saying thank you: to all the contributors, to those who helped shape the ideas and words that made it into print, and to the many who so actively supported the everyday ethics conferences, including Jonathan Tomlinson, Deborah Bowman, Jonathan Drennan and Steph Baker; and for the way we worked together to bring the project to completion. This work included families, friends and colleagues, and those of our blogging patient and service user collaborators, and their networks, and in the wider sense our informal and unpaid/low-paid caring colleagues whom so many of us have worked with and depended on over the years. I also want to thank all those who engage in forms of co-production and write from alternative perspectives; they have contributed in ways they will never know, as Dominic Stenning makes clear. Ideas have histories, and many have paved the way for current models of collaboration, in less welcoming times. The contribution of Peter Beresford to this work has been invaluable. A dedicated text exploring service user, patient and carer experiences of health and care ethics is overdue, as is the critique such perspectives would offer more traditional approaches.

Of course many voices are not here, and they should be, as Tula Brannely points out. We look forward to Ruth de Souza's work, as she contributes distinctively on ethics, diversity and intersectionality. It is pertinent to observe of healthcare ethics that we seem to accept the absence of more diverse ethical perspectives, while working in the most multi-ethnic, multi-cultural and multi-faith communities of practice. The work of Shereen Hussein, Kings College London, was central to our understanding of the vibrant and productive networks of community care workers, from many parts of the world, as they worked through dilemmas and challenges without the resources available to more traditionally educated and employed groups in the health and care workforce. The perspectives of those managing resources and taking organisational decisions are absent too, yet so many of the problems experienced as ethical issues in the preceding chapters can be traced back to resourcing decisions, poor work cultures or mismanagement. Few sympathise with more senior organisational decision makers, still less so the local and national politicians. Yet the key messages of the book mean we cannot simply locate ethics in direct care giving or receiving, or create impermeable boundaries between groups or interests. Understanding ethical practice as that which takes place between people in their decisions, and in systems and processes, means rejecting the individualisation of responsibility while working to understand and analyse broader societal discourses and political decisions. These are all projects for the future.

Finally, the contribution of the only nurse-author in the collection is a reminder of the important and established place of art and creative writing in exploring complex and troubling ideas. I want to thank Molly Case and Rebecca Dunne for sharing their experiences as novices, as they describe the plurality of roles we all inhabit and move through over time. The minutiae of their daily work is grounded in small acts and unspoken concerns, which stay with them over time. So we might begin conversations more often, where our students choose to begin, and be receptive to their disquietude. To echo Suzanne Shale's words, such conversations bring us to questions of how we should live and how we should learn.

Biographies

Hazel Biggs is Professor of Healthcare Law and Bioethics at the University of Southampton. Hazel is also a member of HEAL (the Centre for Health Ethics and Law) at the University of Southampton. She was previously Professor of Medical Law at Lancaster University. Hazel received her first degree from the University of Kent after working for several years as a radiographer and ultrasonographer in the National Health Service. Hazel's research focuses on healthcare law and bioethics generally, with particular emphasis on death and dying and end-of-life decision-making, human reproduction and the beginning of life, and the ethics and law of clinical research. Hazel has published widely on the legal and ethical aspects of each of these areas and has supervised numerous PhD students to completion on related topics. Alongside her university activities, Hazel has chaired local and multi-centre NHS Research Ethics Committees (RECs) and published a book examining the legal and ethical responsibilities of RECs (*Healthcare Research Ethics and Law*) in 2010. She has also been involved with education and training for members of research ethics committees and the medical research community for many years. Hazel was a member of the General Medical Committee (GMC) working group, which in 2010 formulated the guidance Treatment and Care Towards the End of Life: good practice in decision-making. She is currently Editor-in-Chief of *Medical Law Review*, ethics advisor to the Wales Cancer Bank and a Senior Associate of the Royal Society of Medicine.

Tula Brannelly is Lecturer at Bournemouth University. Tula has a long-standing interest in the ethics of care and marginalised groups, and has been involved in mental health research, education and practice, with a strong commitment to co-production and informing change.

Joanne Brown has a background in the social sciences, psychosocial studies and mental health education. She combines academic work with clinical work and is an accredited counsellor and therapist with the British Association for Counselling and Psychotherapy (BACP) and British Psychoanalytic Council (BCP). She has worked in the broad intellectual field of psychosocial studies and psychological therapy for over 25 years, and has a long-standing interest in how clinical learning is contained in an academic context. Her background in psychological therapy informs her questioning of mental health education and the ethical dilemmas which it raises when students might not be training to be therapists, but are being asked to work with insight and a therapeutic use of self. This raises the difficult ethical issues of what might be appropriate boundaries for staff, students and services users, and what kinds of divisions, silencing or holding such boundaries offer when they are drawn. These boundary lines can be challenged for political, personal and educational reasons, and this chapter discusses the author's experience of how she has drawn a boundary line and her reflections on how therapeutic and academic practices or states of mind are in creative tension.

Molly Case is a spoken word artist, writer and nurse, born and brought up in south London. She received a first-class degree in Creative Writing and English Literature from Bath Spa University and during this time spent two years as a care worker looking after people with dementia. Upon leaving Bath, Molly decided to pursue a career in nursing and is currently working at King's College Hospital, London, as a cardiac nurse. In April 2013, she achieved national recognition after performing her poem 'Nursing the Nation' at the Royal College of Nursing, gaining over 350,000 views on YouTube in just a few months. Following this, Molly has performed her poetry up and down the country, across Europe and at Glastonbury Festival. Her debut collection of poetry, *Underneath the Roses Where I Remembered Everything* came out in 2015 with Burning Eye Books. She has appeared in *The Guardian*, The *Independent*, The *Times*, *Elle* magazine and *Huffington Post*, and was named in the Health Service Journal's Inspirational Women list and the BBC's 100 Women list. Molly is a multiple slam winner who was honoured to meet the Queen at Buckingham Palace as part of the Contemporary British Poetry celebrations.

In the next few years, Molly hopes to get poetry into more hospitals by setting up a team of volunteer poets to provide bedside workshops bringing the immediacy of poetic creativity to those who may not have thought about writing before.

Sally Dowling (PhD, PGCert (TLHE), MPH, MA, BSc, RMN) is a Senior Lecturer in the Nursing and Midwifery Department at the University of the West of England (UWE), Bristol. She has worked at UWE since 2009, having previously worked in public health, sexual health and mental health settings. She is a member of the Faculty of Public Health. At UWE, she teaches evidence-based practice and research methods and supervises dissertation students at undergraduate and postgraduate levels, as well as postgraduate research students.

Sally's interest in breastfeeding research came from her own experiences of breastfeeding her youngest two daughters; while they were young, she undertook a PhD at UWE which explored the experiences of women who breastfeed long term. Combined with her public health background, this has led to an interest in a range of other infant feeding issues and, more recently, the practice of sharing breast milk online and via social media. Sally has been exploring this topic and the relating ethical issues through several conference presentations over the past few years and is currently undertaking an analysis of how breast milk sharing and exchange are portrayed in the media (with Dr Aimee Grant, Cardiff University) and co-editing a Special Issue of Maternal and Child Nutrition *Exchanging Breast Milk: From Wet Nursing and Milk Banking to Cross Nursing and Milk Sharing* (with Dr Tanya Cassidy and Prof. Fiona Dykes, University of Central Lancashire), publication due mid-2018. She is particularly interested in how little this issue has been discussed in the UK and whether this is because the ethical issues are different here.

Rebecca Dunne is a Junior Doctor, Peninsula Deanery.

Hilary Engward is a Senior Research Fellow in the Veterans and Families Institute at Anglia Ruskin University, where she leads research into veterans and families living with limb loss. Hilary is a senior lecturer on PhD/EdD courses, with a specific interest in interprofessional learning and working across the medical and health professions. She also teaches healthcare ethics across medical and nursing undergraduate and postgraduate courses at various organisations.

Affiliation: Senior Research Fellow, Veterans and Families Research Institute, Anglia Ruskin University

Marie Ennis-O'Connor, BA is a writer, keynote speaker and digital engagement consultant working with patients, researchers, and healthcare professionals to rediscover the storied heart of medicine. A Stanford Medical School ePatient Scholar, her work with healthcare professionals encourages them to see beyond the biomedical model of disease and to step into the experiential world of patients. She is particularly interested in the concept of 'patient as teacher' and has worked with medical teaching faculties in Ireland, the United States and Australia on programmes to integrate narrative medicine practice in medical education.

Her interest in narrative medicine arose when her she was diagnosed with breast cancer and began writing a blog, Journeying Beyond Breast Cancer, to process the experience. At the time, there was very little written about what happens after treatment ends and she wanted to share her experience with others. She actually realised about a year into writing the blog that her story could provide a unique insight into the long-term impact of cancer.

The kind of information about the lived experience of cancer that she and other bloggers like her were sharing couldn't be found anywhere else. These blogs provide an unparalleled opportunity to develop a richer understanding of what it means to be diagnosed with and live with cancer. In these blogs, you find descriptions of real-time experiences, and she thought that was an incredible gift to researchers and healthcare practitioners.

Her initial enthusiasm for encouraging the use of blogs in research became tempered with a concern about how this information was actually being used, and how she as well as other bloggers, felt about this. She realised the issue was far more complex than she had first thought and that we all need to take a step back and explore the ethical issues associated with using blogs for research.

Angela Fenwick is Associate Professor in Medical Ethics and Education within Medicine at the University of Southampton. She has worked in the Faculty of Medicine since 1995. She co-ordinates the ethics and law theme for the Bachelor of Medicine (BM) undergraduate programmes, as well as teaching research ethics on the postgraduate research courses. From 1993 to 1995, she worked in the School of Education, and from 1995 to 2006 she was Lecturer in Medical Education and instrumental in the design and development of the BM6 and BM4 programmes, as well as contributing to the development of the BM5 programme. From 2002 to 2006, she was the Deputy Director of the BM4 graduate entry programme.

Angela is a member of CELS (Clinical Ethics and Law at Southampton: www.soton.ac.uk/cels), an interdisciplinary group undertaking research and education in the field of clinical ethics and law, with an aim of translating outcomes to a wider community: research and teaching is directed towards the development of national policy and guidelines which improve clinical practice as well as public engagement in the ethical issues which impact on health in society. Her research interests include ethical and legal issues in genetic medicine, the use/abuse of the body in medicine, medical decision-making and the limits of autonomy. Angela set up the Faculty Ethics Committee in 2007 and was the chair of this committee until 2010.

Rebecca Hogue is pursuing a PhD in Health Professions Education from the University of Ottawa, in Ottawa, Canada. She is an Associate Lecturer at the University of Massachusetts–Boston. She holds an MA in Distributed Learning and a BS in computer science. Rebecca is a prolific blogger, currently sharing her academic experiences (http://rjh.goingeast.

ca), her dissertation process (http://livingpathography.org) and her lived experience through breast cancer treatment (http://bcbecky.com). In addition, she and her husband have a travel blog describing their 16-month journey around the world without aeroplanes (http://goingeast.ca). Her research and innovation interests are in the areas of ePatient storytelling (pathography), blogging and online collaboration. Rebecca currently resides in Sunnyvale, California.

Roger Ingham is Professor of Health and Community Psychology within Psychology at the University of Southampton and Director of the Centre for Sexual Health Research. His first degree was awarded by University College London, and his PhD in philosophy, from Oxford University. The Centre for Sexual Health Research has been established for almost 30 years and carries out high-quality research in the field of sexual conduct in the UK and in other countries; it is a multidisciplinary centre, involving a number of disciplines. Research has focused on sexual behaviour among young people, contraception use and decision-making, risk perception, attitudes to services and sex education in school settings, exploring reasons for variations in abortion proportions, parent–child communication about bodies and reproduction, and other related topics. Studies have also been carried out in other European countries, and the Centre coordinated a large Department for International Development (DfID) funded programme of work in developing countries across the world (this programme also involved the Thomas Coram Research Unit at the Institute of Education and the London School of Hygiene and Tropical Medicine, both of the University of London). Professor Ingham has published widely on relevant topics and works closely with policymakers in this country and abroad. He has been for many years a regular advisor/consultant for the World Health Organisation on their reproductive health and AIDS programmes and for other international agencies and was also a member of the former government's Independent Advisory Group for the Teenage Pregnancy Unit and sits on the Teenage Magazine Arbitration Panel. He was a member of the core group involved in the development of the UK National Sexual Health and HIV Strategy.

Andrew Papanikitas is NIHR Academic Clinical Lecturer in General Practice in the Department of Primary Care Health Sciences, and Research Fellow at Harris Manchester College, University of Oxford, UK.

Andrew is an Academic Clinical Lecturer in the Nuffield Department of Primary Care Health Sciences at the University of Oxford. He is a practising medical doctor (GP) in Oxford, with an academic background in history, ethics and education. His PhD thesis was entitled 'From the Classroom to the Clinic: Ethics Education and General Practice'. He has taught medical ethics and law at several UK medical schools, and has published widely on the themes of medical education and medical ethics. He is on the council of the Royal Society of Medicine GP and Primary Healthcare Section and a past president of the Open Section. He is Director for the Society of Apothecaries' Diploma Course in Philosophy and Ethics of Health Care. With John Spicer, he recently edited the *Handbook of Primary Care Ethics* (CRC Press, 2017)

Zoe Picton-Howell PhD, Solicitor (Hons), LLM, LLB (Hons), BA (Hons), Dip RJ (Merit). Her dissertation with honours looked at whether disabled children in the UK have actual rights to education and healthcare (as opposed to 'rights on the books') and concluded they do not.

Her doctoral dissertation for a PhD at Edinburgh Law School takes a legal consciousness theoretical approach and looks at how paediatricians make 'best interest' decisions for severely disabled children.

Zoe was a director of the Scottish Alliance of Child Rights for five years and the Chair of the RCPCH's Parent Advisory Group, as well as a member of the Child Health UK Epilepsy Death Expert Group; the NICE End of Life Care for Infants, Children and Young People Guidelines Committee and the associated Quality Standards Advisory Committee. She also helps NHS England draft child death guidance.

Her interest in the law and ethics related to child health, particularly disabled children's health developed from her experience as Adam Bojelian's (AdsthePoet, http://intheblinkofaneyepoemsbyadambojelian. blogspot.co.uk) mum. As a lawyer with an interest in human rights, I recognised that Adam and his friends simply did not have the rights in real life that they should have had according to international human rights treaties, health professional guidance, statute and case law. She saw huge gaps between what was meant to happen and what actually happened. She also found it fascinating that medics, who held themselves up as being evidence based, often seemed not to look at the evidence when it came to disabled children. For example, they would make assumptions about them rather than looking at available evidence about the child. An example would be that doctors would assume that because Adam had severe physical impairment that he must have severe cognitive impairment despite the fact he was at the top end of the ability range in mainstream school, excelled academically and all this was documented by his school and provided to the medics in the same way it would be for any child. She was also struck that two doctors could see the same child within five minutes but come to completely different conclusions about that child. One day, when Adam was clearly very ill, a consultant reviewed him and said he was absolutely fine, with nothing wrong, and could go home. Five minutes later a second consultant reviewed him and declared him so ill that he needed immediate transfer to intensive care. Adam's condition had not changed in the five minutes. Zoe found it intriguing that two doctors could review the same child and come to such different conclusions. It seemed they must be basing their conclusions on something other than the child. This led to her PhD, which was, in essence, a quest to ask doctors directly what they are doing when making decisions and what part, if any, law, rights and ethics play in those decisions. Her chapter is drawn from the findings of her thesis.

Suzanne Shale is an independent ethics advisor and Visiting Professor at the University College London.

Dominic Stenning After experiencing drug and mental health challenges from a young age, Dominic has been involved with his local trust as a volunteer and independent consultant (non-profit). He is also a member of the East of England Citizens Senate, which was one of the first to be established and continues to lead the way. He was on the steering group of nine 'Experts by Experience' working on The Barker Commission, chaired by economist Dame Kate Barker, which sought to advise government on the future of health & social care. Although The Barker Commission was independent from The Kings Fund, his involvement was initiated through them as a first for patient involvement and set the bar high for including Experts by Experience in the development of such an important report, which he was proud to be a part of. He has worked as an Expert By Experience and a Patient Leader for his trust Cambridgeshire and Peterborough NHS Foundation Trust (CPFT), including Recovery College East, and more recently the trust's Suicide Strategy, which is currently in development. He has spoken at various events and also delivers social media training to staff and patients alike, as he believes this is a vital tool in making things happen. Patient Leaders lead by example, inspire others and affect change through sharing their lived experience combined with the essential leadership skills needed to influence real change as equal partners. Dominic has met some inspirational Patient Leaders and hopes that one day he can inspire others to get involved, as he has done. He has overcome much adversity and has accessed services over much of his lifetime, which has given him valuable insight that he hopes to share with others.

Julie Wintrup teaches health professionals in higher education. Her first qualification as an occupational therapist was followed by many years in community mental health practice and NHS management. She completed an MBA, then a Doctorate in Education and has published research into work-based learning, widening participation, MOOCs, student engagement and ethics education in healthcare. Her teaching, research and scholarly activities centre on the relationship between education, inter/professional development and the 'everyday ethics' of healthcare work. Her teaching interests include mental health, clinical reasoning and decision-making, the role of networks and social media in health, research methods and the pedagogic potential of working with students as co-designers and co-researchers.

David Woods is a Teaching Fellow in Philosophy at the University of Warwick. While studying for his PhD in Philosophy at the University of Southampton, David contributed to teaching on a number of philosophy modules. In 2014, he completed his doctorate. He has won a number of teaching awards.

Index

CPI Antony Rowe
Chippenham, UK
2018-10-16 00:59